hRae

What You Need to Know about ALS

What You Need to Know about ALS

Harry LeVine III

Inside Diseases and Disorders

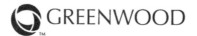
GREENWOOD

An Imprint of ABC-CLIO, LLC
Santa Barbara, California • Denver, Colorado

Library of Congress Cataloging-in-Publication Data

Names: LeVine, Harry, 1949- author.
Title: What you need to know about ALS / Harry LeVine III.
Description: Santa Barbara, California : Greenwood, An Imprint of ABC-CLIO,
  LLC, [2019] | Series: Inside diseases and disorders | Includes
  bibliographical references and index.
Identifiers: LCCN 2019020182 (print) | LCCN 2019020633 (ebook) | ISBN
  9781440863578 (eBook) | ISBN 9781440863561 (hardcopy : alk. paper)
Subjects: LCSH: Amyotrophic lateral sclerosis—Diagnosis. | Amyotrophic
  lateral sclerosis—Treatment. | Amyotrophic lateral
  sclerosis—Complications.
Classification: LCC RC406.A24 (ebook) | LCC RC406.A24 L48 2019 (print) | DDC
  616.8/39—dc23
LC record available at https://lccn.loc.gov/2019020182

ISBN: 978-1-4408-6356-1 (print)
       978-1-4408-6357-8 (ebook)

23 22 21 20 19   1 2 3 4 5

This book is also available as an ebook.

Greenwood
An Imprint of ABC-CLIO, LLC

ABC-CLIO, LLC
147 Castilian Drive
Santa Barbara, California 93117
www.abc-clio.com

This book is printed on acid-free paper ∞

Manufactured in the United States of America

*To Fred Bachmeyer—friend, fellow musician in the
Central Kentucky Concert Band, and
inspiration for writing this book on ALS.*

Contents

Series Foreword

Disease is as old as humanity itself, and it has been the leading cause of death and disability throughout history. From the Black Death in the Middle Ages to smallpox outbreaks among Native Americans to the modern-day epidemics of diabetes and heart disease, humans have lived with—and died from—all manner of ailments, whether caused by infectious agents, environmental and lifestyle factors, or genetic abnormalities. The field of medicine has been driven forward by our desire to combat and prevent disease and to improve the lives of those living with debilitating disorders. And while we have made great strides forward, particularly in the last 100 years, it is doubtful that humankind will ever be completely free of the burden of disease.

Greenwood's Inside Diseases and Disorders series examines some of the key diseases and disorders, both physical and psychological, affecting the world today. Some (such as diabetes, cardiovascular disease, and ADHD) have been selected because of their prominence within modern America. Others (such as Ebola, celiac disease, and autism) have been chosen because they are often discussed in the media and, in some cases, are controversial or the subject of scientific or cultural debate.

Because this series covers so many different diseases and disorders, we have striven to create uniformity across all books. To maximize clarity and consistency, each book in the series follows the same format. Each begins with a collection of 10 frequently asked questions about the disease or disorder, followed by clear, concise answers. Chapter 1 provides a general introduction to the disease or disorder, including statistical information such as prevalence rates and demographic trends. The history of the disease or disorder, including how our understanding of it has evolved over time, is addressed in chapter 2. Chapter 3 examines causes and risk factors, whether genetic, microbial, or environmental, while chapter 4 discusses signs and symptoms. Chapter 5 covers the issues of diagnosis (and misdiagnosis), treatment, and management (whether with drugs, medical procedures, or lifestyle changes). How such treatment, or the lack thereof, affects a patient's long-term prognosis, as well as the risk of complications, are the subject of chapter 6. Chapter 7 explores the disease or disorder's effects on the friends and family of a patient—a dimension often overlooked in discussions of physical and psychological ailments. Chapter 8 discusses prevention strategies, while chapter 9 explores key issues or controversies, whether medical or sociocultural. Finally, chapter 10 profiles cutting-edge research and speculates on how things might change in the next few decades.

Each volume also features five fictional case studies to illustrate different aspects of the book's subject matter, highlighting key concepts and themes that have been explored throughout the text. The reader will also find a glossary of terms and a collection of print and electronic resources for additional information and further study.

As a final caveat, please be aware that the information presented in these books is no substitute for consultation with a licensed health care professional. These books do not claim to provide medical advice or guidance.

Introduction

ALS, or amyotrophic lateral sclerosis, is a rare neuromuscular disease in which muscles controlling movement of the legs, arms, hands, face, jaw, and diaphragm progressively atrophy, leaving the individual unable to stand, use their arms or hands, walk, talk, chew, swallow, and, eventually, breathe. The onset is insidious—a highly localized weakness so subtle that it is often overlooked or a muscle that suddenly stops working. Spreading of muscle weakness and lack of response among connected body regions are hallmarks of ALS, which lead to death over a period averaging 3–5 years. For a few people, the decline is more rapid, in others slower. The physicist Stephen Hawking survived a remarkable 53 years after being told at age 21 that he had only 2 years to live. His story has heartened the ALS field, because it indicates that the disease can be slowed and perhaps someday even stopped.

The primary defect is the degeneration of a specific type of nerve cell, the motor neurons, which control voluntary muscle movement. Other types of neurons such as those responsible for cognition, sensation, and most other mental functions in the brain, sphincter activity, or eye blink do not degenerate. ALS affects primarily middle-aged and older adults, as well as younger individuals who have inheritable forms of the disease. In many ways, it is a mysterious disease with no clear cause in most cases. It only affects voluntary muscles, those controlled by the individual.

The cause(s) of ALS are unknown. Most cases of ALS appear for the first time in a family with no apparent connection to any particular environmental exposure, occupation, or activity, and they are defined as *sporadic*. ALS affects slightly more men than women. About 10 percent of all cases are inherited forms of ALS, genetic mutations in one of a small number of genes for proteins passed along in families. Most individuals carrying one of these mutant genes will develop ALS, frequently at an earlier age than for the sporadic disease. There are no cures for ALS. Currently there are only two therapeutics, which offer a small reduction in functional decline without a significant effect on survival.

Since there are currently no tests for early symptomatic stages that definitively identify ALS, diagnosis is a process of excluding other diseases that present similar symptoms; these diseases are treatable and generally have more favorable outcomes. The process is lengthy, in part because progression is a primary characteristic of ALS and is required for a solid diagnosis. While direct causation is difficult to prove, the most striking risk factors for ALS are military service, particularly active duty in U.S. armed forces in conflict zones, athletes and highly physically fit individuals, as well as some industrial and agricultural exposures. This has implications for individuals with military service and for the Veterans Administration (VA), which has taken the responsibility of caring for veterans with ALS.

Treatment is primarily symptomatic, providing assistance as patients' physical ability to move and take care of themselves declines. This includes treating pain in immobilized joints and symptoms, such as excess salivation. Maintaining the patient's weight while their ability to eat and swallow without choking is impaired becomes challenging. Combining the loss of the patient's ability to talk and otherwise communicate creates additional stress on the caregivers, who are primarily a spouse or another family member. The need for care for the caregivers, who are also facing the loss of a loved one, is finally being recognized.

ALS has been brought to public attention by high-profile individuals with ALS, such as the physicist Stephen Hawking, the baseball player Lou Gehrig, and a number of other athletes. The ALS Ice Bucket Challenge, an online phenomenon, went viral and attracted interest and support, including significant funding that has driven research in new directions. Potential therapies based on different patient-derived, stem-cell-based approaches and antisense oligonucleotides that prevent a specific disease-causing protein from being produced are now making their way toward clinical trials.

Essential Questions

1. WHAT CAUSES ALS?

In most cases of ALS, the cause is unknown (sporadic). You can't "catch" ALS by being exposed to someone with ALS because it is noninfectious. In about 10 percent of ALS patients, the cause is a change in the DNA coding (gene) for the production of one of a small number of proteins. The altered protein causes the selective dysfunction and death of certain motor neurons controlling the muscles that move the arms, legs, hands, and the diaphragm, which powers breathing.

2. WHO IS MOST LIKELY TO SUFFER FROM ALS?

Risk factors for ALS have been difficult to identify, but middle age, service in the military, exposure to environmental pollution, jobs in mining or exposure to toxins, and high-intensity athletics like football, especially with repeated head trauma, show statistically significant association with the sporadic form of the disease. These aren't strictly considered causes, as these activities affect individuals differently and most people exposed to them do not develop ALS.

3. DOES ALS RUN IN FAMILIES?

If more than one person in a family of genetically related individuals has ALS, there is a good chance that the disease is genetically inherited (runs in the family). This form of the disease is designated as familial ALS (fALS). There is a 50 percent chance that a child born to someone with fALS will inherit the mutant gene and in many cases will develop ALS. Not all genes that can cause ALS are known at this time. Roughly 10 percent of all ALS cases are fALS and carry a genetic mutation in an ALS gene.

4. HOW IS ALS DIAGNOSED?

ALS is diagnosed by starting with a clinical history and a series of neurological examinations, including electrophysiological, neuroimaging, and clinical laboratory testing with neuropathologic examinations, if appropriate, to rule in or rule out ALS. When there is an absence of electrophysiological and neuroimaging evidence of ALS but there is clinical laboratory evidence of other medical conditions whose symptoms are similar to ALS, this suggests that a different disease is present. Progression is a characteristic feature of ALS, so repeat clinical and electrophysiological examinations at least six months apart are performed in order to assess spreading and changes in severity.

5. WHAT ARE THE EARLY SYMPTOMS OF ALS?

Early symptoms of ALS include localized muscle weakness, muscle wasting, or lack of response in trying to move a limb; spasticity or hyperresponsive reflexes are suggestive of ALS. Progressive spread of these symptoms to connected regions of the musculature is a key indication of ALS.

6. WHAT ARE THE SYMPTOMS OF ALS AS IT PROGRESSES?

ALS selectively affects neurons that communicate with voluntary muscle movement in the arms and legs; the diaphragm, which controls breathing; as well the face and jaw for talking and chewing, and the throat for swallowing. Nerves controlling the muscles of the heart, sphincter control, and eye movement are not affected, for unknown reasons. As the disease progresses, weakness or wasting (atrophy) and lack of response for movement spread from an initial focal site to involve nearby regions. Eventually ALS patients lose the ability to stand, walk, use their arms or hands, chew, swallow, and talk, until their diaphragm weakens enough to prevent breathing on their own and they require artificial breathing assistance. A subgroup of ALS patients also display signs of behavioral disturbance, emotional and personality changes, and language impairment, which complicate caregiving.

7. HOW IS ALS TREATED?

Because there is presently no cure for ALS, the symptoms are treated to minimize discomfort and to maintain function as long as possible. Assistive technology is provided to accommodate the loss of mobility and ability to communicate, and noninvasive ventilation assists with breathing.

Two medications, riluzole and edavarone, have received Federal Drug Administration (FDA) approval for treatment of ALS, although their effects on the progression rate, severity, and increase in survival time are moderate at best and the efficacy differs between individuals.

8. IS ALS A PAINFUL DISEASE?

The nerves that degenerate in ALS are motor neurons that activate muscle activity. The nerves that register pain are not affected in ALS. However, stiffening of muscles that no longer contract, spasms of the muscles whose controlling nerves are degenerating, and shortening of muscles as they atrophy cause pain in joints that no longer can straighten. Uncontrolled muscle spasms can also be painful.

9. WHAT DO ALS PATIENTS DIE FROM?

Most ALS patients die when their diaphragm muscles lose the neuronal control of their ability to contract and relax to move air in and out of the lungs. Many patients use noninvasive ventilation to assist breathing for a period of time, and some opt for a surgically emplaced tube powered by a ventilator. Difficulties with chewing and swallowing, from the loss of control of muscles of the jaw and throat, often lead to choking, which can cause aspiration of material into the lungs, followed by pneumonia. The majority of ALS patients die in their sleep.

10. WHAT RESEARCH IS BEING DONE?

Finding and developing new biomarkers to speed the diagnosis of ALS, to follow its early progression, and to report on the effectiveness of therapeutic interventions are the focus of a number of research groups. These include biofluid tests (blood and cerebrospinal fluid) as well as imaging and improved noninvasive ways to measure changes in muscle and motor neuron function.

The advancement of the ability to study stem cells, nonspecialized cells isolated from fat or bone marrow, has opened new ways to understand similarities and differences between familial and sporadic ALS. Future plans include testing transplanted stem cells or their secreted products as therapeutics in clinical trials. In cases of familial ALS where the mutated protein is known, agents such as antisense oligonucleotides are targeting the damaged gene or its product.

1

What Is ALS?

It starts with muscle weakness in the arms, hands, legs, or feet that often is ignored by the individual. Instead of going away, the weakness becomes more profound over a period of weeks to months and expands from an initially small region to the whole limb. Some people develop stiffness or muscle twitches (fasciculations) as the control of muscles in the face and neck becomes compromised, spreading beyond to muscles that regulate swallowing, chewing, and speaking and that also control facial expressions. They suffer excessively strong reflex responses without apparent cause. Virtually all voluntary muscles, muscles that require the brain to send them a signal to contract, are susceptible to the inexorable progression of the symptoms. Involuntary muscle types, like the heart muscle, which does not require brain activation to beat, are unaffected in ALS. Certain voluntary muscles, such as those governing sphincters and eye movement, for some unknown reason remain unaffected.

As ALS progresses, the weakness that began in an extremity or on one side of the body becomes more generalized, spreading to larger and larger areas and eventually affecting both left and right sides of the body. The muscles of the diaphragm that control breathing become weaker and weaker, leading to paralysis of the diaphragm and death in the majority of ALS patients. Breathing difficulties combined with head and neck muscular weakness make it difficult to swallow and result in increasing instances of choking, in which food or liquids enter the lungs, causing aspiration pneumonia, the other major cause of death in ALS.

At the core of ALS, the primary disease specifically manifests in specific neuronal cells, which connect the part of the brain called the *motor cortex*, responsible for voluntary movement and conscious action, with the associated muscles. The clinical name of the disease, amyotrophic (muscle wasting or atrophy/shrinking) lateral sclerosis (degeneration of the lateral nerves, the pathways that extend down the sides of the spinal nerve column), describes the symptoms. Most people in the United States refer to ALS as Lou Gehrig's disease, named after a famous baseball player whose playing career was prematurely ended at age thirty-six by the disease and who died shortly thereafter. In Europe and other parts of the world, it is known as motor neuron disease. The naming is unfortunate and causes some confusion because the category of motor neuron diseases includes a constellation of nerve-muscle diseases with different mechanisms and outcomes that can be distinguished from ALS, many of which can be effectively treated.

THE NERVOUS SYSTEM

The brain is divided internally into regions containing neurons that are interconnected to perform specific functions, and certain regions are connected to serve more general purposes. These regional divisions are generally not distinguishable to the unaided eye. The German neuropathologist Korbinian Brodmann defined 43 regions containing different types of cells in 1909 by staining thinly sliced sections of brain obtained at autopsy with colored dyes and viewing through a microscope. In 2016, magnetic resonance imaging (MRI) of living brain in human subjects defined 180 separate regions distinguishable by their activation states during different tasks.

ALS does not affect all kinds of nerves. For reasons that are currently unknown, nerves responsible for sensation (heat, cold, pain, taste, touch), which do not reside in the motor cortex but whose axons (connecting fiber of a nerve) also extend along the spinal cord like motor neurons do, are unaffected. Although uncontrolled muscle cramps and overactive reflexes can be painful, ALS patients, in general, are relatively spared the pain of some disease states that more directly involve or impact sensory nerves.

The Neighborhood: Other Cell Types

Although the degeneration and death of motor neurons is a prominent feature of ALS, it is clear that other cell types play critical roles in the disease process. This is often called the *neighborhood involvement* of multiple cell types in the process. In animal models of genetic forms of ALS in which the mutation of certain proteins drives the disease, the expression of the mutant protein in the motor neuron is critical in the onset and early stages. Expression of the mutant protein in nonneuronal cells also seems to be required to modulate the disease progression. In the brain and spinal column, several types of nonnerve glial cells that nurture neurons envelop the motor neuron cell bodies, the long neuronal processes, and the nerve endings called *synapses*, which connect with muscle cells and therefore are involved in ALS.

Astrocytes are one type of nonnerve glial cell that performs supportive functions in the nervous system. Under normal conditions, these special cells provide protection from toxic accumulation of neurotransmitters and contribute physical support and growth factors to maintain the health of the neurons, as well as that of the synaptic endings of the motor neurons contacting individual muscle fibers. Other cell types like microglia, the resident white blood cells of the brain, and their cousins, the tissue macrophages, also a white blood cell type, can become dysfunctional and contribute to the progression of ALS. Their normal function is as a cellular component of the immune system in the brain and other tissues, respectively, responsible for removing infectious agents and toxic materials and debris from their environment.

Both astrocytes and microglia/macrophages respond to their environment, producing and responding to a variety of signaling molecules depending on conditions, especially the state of the neuronal cells. This complex network is disrupted in ALS, when neurons start displaying alarm signals as they become dysfunctional. The astrocytes and microglia respond in turn to the situation in ways that would be helpful in nondisease situations, but in the disrupted state of the neurons, these glial responses further exacerbate the neuronal dysfunction and contribute to the motor neuron demise. Some of these factors also affect the muscle cells and their communication with the motor neurons, resulting in a spiral of toxic insults and responses.

THE DEGENERATIVE PROCESS IN ALS

Both neurons and muscles are affected in ALS. Both cell types degenerate as the disease progresses. It is not completely clear whether the same processes are driving degeneration in both cell types, except perhaps in some of the genetic inherited forms of ALS. It is possible that some of the ALS disease subtypes result from differences in dominance among the multiple factors driving the disease in one or the other cell types as well as the impact of neighboring glial cells.

Motor Nerve Dysfunction

The motor pathways affected in ALS start in the motor cortex. Two main nerve tracts are affected. Upper motor neurons, in the motor cortex of the brain, connect with motor neurons in the base of the brain that send their processes to connect with muscles in the head, neck, and face and to lower motor neurons in the spinal cord. One-third of the cases of ALS primarily involve these upper motor neurons. This form of ALS is defined as *bulbar ALS*, named after the region of affected neurons in the base of the brain.

The remaining two-thirds of classic ALS cases, defined as *spinal ALS*, primarily involve a second set of motor neurons that extend from the motor cortex all the way down the spinal cord; they connect with other sets of motor neurons that make contact with the muscles controlling arm and leg movement. The initial presentation of the particular pattern of the loss of muscular control and eventual atrophy of the disconnected muscles in ALS depends on which of these sets of neurons degenerate first. These different forms of ALS have different prognoses (probable outcome) and rates of progression, although both are inevitably fatal. Individuals can also develop variable combinations of the bulbar and spinal forms of ALS.

Voluntary Muscle Dysfunction

The region of contact between the motor neuron and the muscle fiber that it controls is called a *neuromuscular synapse*. Within this synapse, a number of biochemical processes are disturbed in ALS, which eventually results in breakdown and dysfunction of this critical neuromuscular connection. In addition to and as a result of the defective connection, muscle metabolism, strength, and contractile mechanism are damaged, causing muscle atrophy. The nature of the changes in ALS in the contact zone between the motor neuron and the muscle fiber called the *neuromuscular junction* are unlike those caused by trauma or other kinds of neuromuscular damage.

The neuromuscular junction is a cooperative venture of the motor neuron, the muscle fiber, and a special kind of glial cell called a *terminal Schwann cell*, which is critical to forming and maintaining a stable neuromuscular junction. The disassembly of this tripartite connection and resultant loss of neuronal connectivity and muscle activation leads to ALS clinical symptoms and degeneration of the muscle cell.

The major glial cells outside of the brain are called *Schwann cells*, one type of which produces the insulating protein-lipid complex myelin. These myelinating Schwann cells are responsible for enwrapping lower motor neurons to maintain their size and promote conduction of the action potential, the signal conveyed by the nerve to the muscle. The terminal

Schwann cell lacks the myelin but is crucial for the development, maintenance, and regeneration of the neuromuscular synapse. Little is understood about how these cells are involved in initiating the pathology of ALS, but they are known under some conditions to switch from a maintenance state to an activated regenerating state, in which they remove degraded axons and other cellular debris from degenerating neurons. They also produce vital growth and maintenance factors for both neurons and muscle cells. Overactivation of these terminal Schwann cells leads to their death, which reduces the effectiveness of reinnervation of muscle fibers by nearby sprouting motor neuron termini.

While it is generally accepted that ALS is a disease that primarily affects motor neurons, it is clear that other cell types, especially those in proximity to the affected neurons, play key roles in the neuromuscular degeneration, but the magnitude of this neighborhood effect remains to be established. Genetic forms of the disease seem to begin in the motor neurons, while the effects of those same genes in other cell types seem to modulate the progression of the disease. A controversy that remains to be resolved is whether ALS is better described as *dying forward*, beginning in the motor neurons, or as a *dying back* process that begins at the neuromuscular junction and progresses back to the motor neuron cell body, causing its death. There is evidence for both mechanisms, so there remains the possibility that both processes could be going on simultaneously, or differentially, depending on the specific inciting process(es).

THE ROLE OF GENETICS IN ALS

Like many complex human diseases, ALS is influenced by a multifaceted web of genetic components that play a role in inheritance and expression of susceptibility to the disease. An individual inherits a copy of each gene from each parent. Some gene mutations are expressed in a dominant fashion in family members, which means that an individual only needs to receive a single copy of the mutant gene from one parent to display the mutant trait, in this case the susceptibility to ALS. These mutations occur among a small number of certain genes and lead with high probability to development of ALS. The age of symptom onset for an individual depends both on the identity of the gene and on the specific mutation in that gene. These mutations are relatively rare, comprising 5–10 percent of all cases of ALS, and they are usually associated with a younger age of symptom onset compared to the 90–95 percent of other ALS cases. The other cases are considered sporadic because they are not linked to a detectable genetic change. The dominant genetic mutations have been valuable in producing animal models of ALS in order to learn about mechanisms and to test potential therapeutic strategies.

Not all mutations in a gene lead to a noticeable effect on their own. Some subtly affect how much and when the gene product is produced or cause only a minor change in the properties of the product. Modern gene sequencing technology makes possible large-scale analysis of the connection of slight changes (variants) in gene sequences with some observable change or susceptibility to a disease. The changes are inherited in offspring but have insufficient impact on their own to cause a noticeable effect. Genome-wide association studies (GWAS) of these minor genetic changes make it possible to determine which changes in multiple genes are connected (associated) with the disease state, although individually they would not cause disease. This is important information because it indicates which gene products and their molecular pathways interact with one another to increase the probability of producing the disease state. These genetic variants can significantly alter the process and age of onset of ALS.

At the level of the gene, an additional level of control that does not affect the DNA sequence itself consists of modifications in the way a gene is expressed (turned on or off) based on previous experiences. These modifications, called *epigenetic effectors*, are modifications of the basic chromosome structure that can reflect life experiences by altering gene expression. Their effects can even skip generations to have profound effects. Generally, epigenetic changes are not transmitted to the next generation, but there are some notable exceptions. The connection of epigenetic regulation to ALS remains to be established, but its prevalence in other disease states suggests that it could provide additional information on the disease.

THE SPECTRUM OF ALS

At first, ALS was considered a single disease, a set of symptoms describing a specific unhealthy condition, even though multiple motor neuron diseases affecting nerve-muscle function were recognized by physicians. Over the years since its 19th-century description and naming by Jean-Martin Charcot, the number of apparently different diseases sharing a similar constellation of symptoms grew until it was gradually accepted by neurologists that ALS was not a single disease.

ALS Is a Syndrome

ALS is, in fact, not only a syndrome but a collection of syndromes, a set of clinical conditions that affect different groups of common symptoms in individuals, all culminating in paralysis and atrophy of voluntary muscles. The differences in the groups of symptoms are particularly significant to caregivers because they distinguish symptomatic trajectories, symptom-atology, and prognoses, although the final outcome is the same. These syn-dromes significantly stand apart from other motor neuron diseases with other distinctive features and prognoses.

The grouping of ALS into half-dozen variants provides some consist-ency in symptoms and prognosis. Some of the variants are relatively rare, while others represent the majority of the cases.

Incidence and Prevalence

Incidence and prevalence are two slightly different ways of looking at how often disease occurs in a population and what fraction of that popula-tion is living with the disease. Incidence is the rate of *new* cases of disease per 100,000 population over a time period. Prevalence is the number of cases *still alive* as a fraction of the total population at risk over a time per-iod, usually a year. Given these statistics, a simple calculation predicts that the average primary care physician in the United States will see one ALS case in their professional lifetime.

Although there are few true population-based studies outside of Eur-ope, it is clear that there are differences in prevalence between African Americans, Native Americans, Hispanics, and non-Hispanic groups of European descent. In both the United States and Europe, the incidence of ALS is 1–2 new cases per 100,000 people. In the European population as well as in populations of European descent, the prevalence is 2.6–3.0 cases per 100,000 people, and the lifetime risk in European populations is 1 in 350 for men and 1 in 400 for women. Thus, in European ancestral popula-tions, ALS is 1.2–1.5 times more common in men than in women. Popula-tions with mixed ancestral origin have lower rates of incidence and prevalence than those of European ancestry.

Age of Onset

Despite being overall a relatively rare disease, ALS is the most common neurodegenerative disease of midlife. In European populations, the most common (median) age of onset is 65 years, although the average age is closer to the midfifties. These ages of onset have not changed materially across population-based registers of cases. The recent recognition that there is a continuum between ALS and frontotemporal dementia (FTD), which affects cognition and behavior, has altered the ways that people are included in registers of disease incidence. This has resulted in changes in the statis-tics that now show an apparent increase in ALS risk in later stages of life.

Prognosis

Unfortunately, prognosis in ALS has not substantially improved, and survival remains at 3–5 years postdiagnosis, depending on the variant of ALS. Some of the so-called restricted forms of ALS, which constitute 10 percent or less of all ALS cases, can live for up to 10 or more years after diagnosis. Riluzole and edaravone, the current Food and Drug Administration (FDA)–approved pharmacological treatments to extend life span and functionality, have had little impact, with effect sizes of increasing survival on the order of a few months for riluzole. The effects of edaravone on survival have not been determined. Palliative treatments providing symptomatic relief and improvements in the quality of life are relatively successful, but they do not appreciably extend patient life once symptoms have begun.

ALS VARIANTS

ALS symptoms involve the loss of function of voluntary muscle groups developing over a period of weeks to months. Any voluntary muscle can be affected, resulting in a great variety of presentations, such as loss of control of speech, foot drop (weakness), or localized paralysis. The initial onset of loss of muscle control is focal and confined to one side of the body. It then spreads, first within that body region and then into other regions served by the same nerve connections. Eventually the disease spreads to other body regions, affecting muscles controlled by motor neurons.

There is no one single definitive diagnostic test for ALS. Differential diagnoses are arrived at for each individual patient. It is, however, particularly important to establish which form of ALS is present, to the best of the ability of the diagnostic team. Understanding the form of the disease gives some sense of the rate of progression, which permits managing care for the patient to relieve symptoms and maximize the quality of life. It is also important to establish whether other diseases with some of the same symptoms as ALS are present, because a number of them can be successfully treated to restore a normal or near-normal life span and recovery of function.

Classic ALS

Classic ALS symptoms and outcomes that mirror the original description of the disease account for 70 percent of the ALS cases diagnosed. Two-thirds of these classic cases are the spinal variant, initially usually concentrated on one side of the body. At first, the facial muscles are spared, which distinguishes the spinal variant from the other classic ALS type: the bulbar form.

Accounting for about 30 percent of the remaining classical cases, bulbar ALS derives its name from the part of the brain called the *brain stem*, a bulbous region at the base of the brain from which the spinal cord extends. This brain stem region is where neurons from the brain motor cortex make connections with the upper motor neurons that control voluntary muscle activity in the head, neck, and face. Loss of bulbar neuron control results in jaw spasticity; distorted facial expressions; tongue wasting; fasciculations; difficulty in chewing, swallowing, and talking; and other signs of loss of bulbar innervation. Symptoms eventually spread to the limbs and other parts of the body initially affected in the spinal form of classical ALS.

ALS–Frontotemporal Dementia (ALS-FTD)

The regions of the brain that are involved in the cognitive functions, such as memory, planning, language, and behavior, were traditionally considered to be essentially unaffected in ALS. Over the past 20 years, however, with more sensitive diagnostic procedures, a significant proportion—approximately 15–20 percent—of ALS cases have specific progressive cognitive impairment and behavioral changes that fulfill the diagnostic criteria for *frontotemporal dementia* in addition to the motor symptoms. The combination causes significant additional burden on caregivers. Patient apathy and loss of sympathy for others are the most commonly affected behaviors.

Autopsy studies have identified the basis for the clinical observations for FTD and ALS-FTD as the development of deposits of the protein TDP43 inside neurons and the degeneration of the frontal and temporal brain regions responsible for specific aspects of cognition and behavior. These protein deposits are highly similar to the pathological deposits of the same protein found in frontotemporal dementia, also known as Pick's disease. While FTD by itself also affects behaviors such as poor judgement and mood changes, it eventually leads to full dementia, which is rarely observed in ALS.

Isolated Bulbar Involvement

Also known as pseudobulbar palsy or isolated bulbar palsy, about 5 percent of ALS patients show only bulbar symptoms for years without spreading to other regions (unlike bulbar-onset ALS). Patients with this form of

ALS are mostly women, who suffer spastic speech control and commonly display emotional liability.

Restricted Phenotypes of ALS

Classic ALS usually eventually spreads to affect both lower and upper motor neurons and their associated muscle groups. A number of different restricted presentations of ALS individually account for small proportions of ALS cases. One group accounting for about 5 percent of the classic cases affects only lower motor neurons (progressive muscular atrophy) or only upper motor neurons (primary lateral sclerosis). These patients survive significantly longer than those with classic ALS and can live for more than 10 years or even reach full life expectancy.

Rare Phenotypes of ALS

These forms of ALS are rare in total, accounting for only 3 percent of ALS cases. *Cachexia* is a wasting weakening condition, manifesting as a dramatic loss of weight with no assignable explanation. It can evolve into classic ALS with upper or lower motor neuron involvement, or both. A form of ALS with very poor prognosis is *initial respiratory onset*, with weakness of the diaphragm and flexor neck muscles that stabilize the neck. Weakness of the diaphragm and the resultant respiratory failure is usually a late-stage development and the cause of death of many ALS patients.

This chapter covered the basic biology of the neuromuscular system and the effects of ALS on its function and described multiple different types of ALS and the ways that they differ from one another. The incidence and prevalence of the occurrence of ALS indicates that ALS is a rare disease. At the same time, it is the most common neurodegenerative disease of midlife. We will next follow the history of the recognition and unification of the group of muscle wasting diseases now known as ALS. An overview of the current understanding of the mechanism of the disease process and consideration of the hurdles to finding a cure will provide some appreciation for the difficulties in developing treatments that alter the progression of the disease.

2

The History of ALS

Before the 19th century, without a clear understanding of how the brain and its control of muscle activity operated, physicians were helpless to confront a confusing set of muscle-wasting conditions that mysteriously and suddenly appeared in a small area of an arm, leg, shoulder, or jaw. The area of the original weakness enlarged and spread relentlessly, causing death within a few years. Finally, in 1874 the commonalities among cases were recognized, and the disease was given the name *amyotrophic lateral sclerosis*. It was observed that family members could also develop the muscle wasting, which suggested a hereditary component to the disease. The baffling multiple forms that the disease can take, including an originally unrecognized association with another disease called *frontotemporal dementia*, and the spread among muscles connected by the same nerves made it difficult to treat. Many hurdles still lie in the way of effectively treating ALS. Slowly, these impediments are being overcome, and clinical trials of potential therapeutics are being carried out, although so far they have been largely disappointing.

ALS AS A MOTOR NEURON DISEASE

In the middle of the 19th century, in Europe and the United States while physiologists were trying to understand what the nervous system was comprised of and how it worked to convey sensation and muscular movement, clinicians were becoming increasingly baffled by their patients' symptoms. They were seeing more and more conditions with symptoms of progressive muscle weakness and wasting or atrophy of muscles spreading with no apparent relationship to a physical injury. They were hampered in their ability to treat these conditions because they had little concept of how the nervous system was interconnected and how that was related to what was going wrong. In the mid-1800s, clinical examination skills were poorly developed, and none of today's diagnostic armamentarium was available. The discovery of X-rays was 50 years away, and magnetic resonance imaging was almost 125 years in the future. It was not until the 1980s that ion channels, the proteins that conduct ionic currents, and neurotransmitter receptors that respond to the chemical signals crossing the synaptic gaps between nerve cells and muscle cells were identified. The diagnostic value of overactive tendon reflexes and other symptoms of ALS recognized today was not appreciated.

Most importantly, there was no accepted way of parsing the multitude of clinical observations into different disease states linked by common features so that they could be approached logically. A number of French and English neurologists began to use symptomatic observations to classify nerve and muscle disorders by whether they were primarily due to nerve diseases or muscle diseases. This turned out to be difficult to do in practice. The first description of a case of ALS was provided by Charles Bell (1774–1842) in 1824. In 1850, the neurologist François Aran (1817–1861) described a series of 11 cases with different configurations of muscular weakness and limb atrophy, calling them *progressive muscular atrophy*. Importantly, he recognized that not all muscles were affected, only certain ones.

Although his lumping of cases turned out many years later to be variants of ALS rather than "classical" ALS, Aran's analysis set the stage for further organization of diseases of muscle weakness and atrophy. Up to this point, these diseases were defined by their clinical (symptomatic) presentation. What was missing was the connection at autopsy with anatomical changes that could be linked to the symptoms.

Newly developed techniques for staining tissue to reveal nervous-system-structure changes began to provide evidence that suggested causation. In 1859, Louis Dumenil (1823–1890) described a form of muscle weakness that primarily affected muscles in the face and neck. Pathological analysis showed degeneration of upper motor neurons running from the motor cortex of the brain to the affected regions. In 1874, after more than a decade of intense study, the French neurologist Jean-Martin Charcot (1825–1893) used missing or degenerating neurons connected to the affected muscles as part of the clinicopathological description of the disease he called *amyotrophic lateral sclerosis*. He recognized that the symptomatology took multiple forms but chose to describe the prototypic case in order to provide clarity in what had previously been a muddle. Naming the syndrome was a key step in the study of ALS.

WHAT'S IN A NAME: THE CLINICAL IMPORTANCE OF NAMING A DISEASE

Why is a name important? Many talented neurologists described essential clinical and pathological features of ALS in multiple patients, but they did not give a name to the disorder they were studying. A name is a defining characteristic that can be used to recognize and promote understanding of a syndrome, which is a condition that can be characterized by a set of associated symptoms. Done properly, naming a condition can facilitate understanding and promote progress. Understanding the biology can establish root causes, but this is more successful when applied to a set of cases that share critical characteristics. Similar biology can give rise to different clinical characteristics. Naming a set of clinical characteristics as a disease helps clinicians decide on treatments. William Gowers (1854–1915) defined stages of ALS and was the first to discuss the potential for treatments and the lack of efficacy of treatments current at the time. He proposed many of the treatments that are in use today, such as controlling salivation and considering dietary changes. He also discussed liquid feeding through a nasalgastric (NG) tube when patients were unable to swallow properly.

Today, unfortunately, we still have to rely almost solely on clinical symptoms to diagnose ALS and prove it by autopsy. Progress has been slow on identifying valid biomarkers for ALS, particularly readily accessible biomarkers in body fluids such as blood. This is a major impediment to finding effective therapies, since as has been recognized for multiple neurodegenerative diseases, symptomatic neurodegenerative disease is already a late-stage disease, frequently more difficult or impossible to treat effectively. This topic will be covered in more detail in chapter 4.

By giving the disease a name, Charcot created a reference point for others to begin to search for explanations for causes and for treatments that would help their patients. No longer was ALS an incomprehensible, seemingly random morass of disparate observations and symptoms. In connecting clinical observations with pathological changes in nerves and muscles, there was now a pathway to the search for causes and earlier diagnosis. Although Charcot purposely simplified the criteria for the condition, he was describing an archetype to which the details of individual cases could be compared. By doing so, he provided a paradigm for diagnosis and a target for further research. Classical ALS describes most—some 70 percent—of the cases; the nonclassical forms appear as variants with different symptoms of the disease accompanying the core set of classical ALS symptoms.

Understanding what was causing ALS and what was happening in the patient during disease progression continued to develop after Charcot established the connection between the symptoms and changes in neuromuscular function that characterized the group of diseases he defined as the ALS syndrome. Two versions of ALS that affected isolated body regions were later described: the flail arm variant by Alfred Vulpian (1826–1887) in 1886 and the flail leg variant by Pierre Marie (1853–1940) in 1918. In 1945, U.S. naval physicians described a mysterious outbreak of a neuromuscular disease similar to ALS but including symptoms of Parkinson's disease and dementia among the Chamorro inhabitants on the island of Guam. Named *ALS-Parkinson-dementia* in 1956, it may have been a result of a toxin in seeds of a cycad plant (e.g., Ginkgo) in their diet. Incidence decreased with lower cycad seed consumption.

EVOLUTION IN DIAGNOSIS

During the 1950s, evaluation of electrodiagnostic testing of both muscle and nerve function began in cases of clinically suspected cases of ALS. In 1969, Edward H. Lambert (1915–2003) published the first electrodiagnostic criteria for ALS diagnosis. The first clinical scale for ALS diagnosis, the ALS–Clinical Functional Rating Scale (ALSFRS) based on activities of daily living, was established in 1996 with a revision (ALSFRS-R) in 1999 to include respiratory criteria. The need for accepted standards for diagnosing ALS for clinical trials was clear. The World Federation of Neurology met in 1990 to work out standards, which were published as the El Escorial criteria in 1994. Subsequent Airlie House criteria revisions published in 2000, to which the Awaji electrodiagnostic criteria were added in 2008, define current standards for clinical trials.

DRUG APPROVAL

The first drug approved for ALS by the FDA in the United States was riluzole in 1995, followed by approvals in Europe in 1996 and in Japan in 1998. The second and, as of 2018, the only other drug approved for ALS treatment was edaravone, which was approved in 2015 in Japan and South Korea, followed by U.S. FDA approval in 2017.

DISCOVERY OF NEUROPATHOLOGY AND DISEASE MECHANISMS

The first gene mutation found to cause an inherited version of ALS (fALS) was SOD1 coding for the enzyme superoxide dismutase-1, discovered in 1993. This mutant gene was used soon after in 1994 to create the first mouse animal model of ALS, which reproduced major characteristics of the human disease. Other major fALS mutant genes have been identified. Another protein, TDP43, the protein coded by the TARDBP gene was found clumped in motor neurons in both ALS and frontotemporal dementia in 2006.

In 2008, TARDBP mutants were also found to cause genetic forms of ALS. Also in 2008, FUS (fused-in-sarcoma) mutants were shown to be a genetic cause of ALS. In 2011, the C9ORF72 gene was identified as being the most common genetic cause of ALS. Although only about 10 percent of all ALS cases are of genetic origin, the genes have proved useful in learning about cellular changes that can lead to the disease. By 2018, more than 20 SOD1, 12 FUS, a number of c9ORF72, and several less common fALS gene mouse models had been produced.

So far, clinical trials of drug candidates in humans have largely failed to show the efficacy that was observed in the fALS animal models, primarily the SOD1 model, used in preliminary testing. so understanding the differences in the disease process between humans and the animal models remains an issue.

GIVING ALS A FACE

Just as a name for a disease increases recognition of the condition among physicians, having a famous and widely recognized person with the disease exemplifies the disease for the general public. Although Charcot first defined ALS in 1874, since it was a rare disease with patients who did not survive beyond a few years, families and patients generally suffered in anonymity. In the United States, to get the attention of a public audience, ALS had to strike a sports hero: the New York Yankees baseball player Lou Gehrig, in the late 1930s. The national shock was such that after his death only 2 years after his diagnosis, ALS became commonly known in the United States as Lou Gehrig's disease.

Lou Gehrig

Henry Louis "Lou" Gehrig (June 19, 1903–June 2, 1941) was first baseman for the New York Yankees baseball team for 17 seasons during the

1920s and 1930s, playing 2,130 consecutive games until he took himself out of a game in 1939 due to the effect of deteriorating strength and coordination on his performance. His batting average had dropped from 0.343 to 0.143, and he was unable to run the bases without stumbling. Far from the "Iron Horse" moniker he had earned from his longevity and power hitting, Gehrig could now barely hit the ball out of the infield.

Examination at the Mayo Clinic revealed that Gehrig had ALS. On his 36th birthday, he was told his diagnosis and was given up to 3 years to live. He accepted his diagnosis stoically, determined to carry on as long as he could. On June 21, 1939, he made a short, emotional retirement speech in front of a packed Yankee stadium crowd, telling them, "Today I consider myself the luckiest man on the face of the earth." Gehrig received many honors and awards and was the first major league baseball player to have his jersey number (four) retired. He continued to decline physically although he remained mentally sharp. Lou Gehrig died at home on June 2, 1941.

Stephen Hawking

The English theoretical physicist and cosmologist Stephen William Hawking (December 9, 1942–March 14, 2018) is recognized for his contributions to general relativity theory, gravitational theory, and the behavior of cosmic phenomena of black holes, as well as for bringing science to a wider audience. As a child, he was interested in science, particularly in the sky and the stars. With an IQ of 160, he was bright but bored, and he did not do well in school. In 1963 when Hawking was a 21-year-old graduate student, he was diagnosed with ALS, known in England as motor neuron disease, and was given 2½ years to live. That deadline caused him to buckle down and focus on his doctoral work in cosmology.

He never looked back. In 1969, already well past his predicted survival, he yielded and began to use a wheelchair instead of crutches. The progression of his disability slowed down over the years, and he continued to live and work, slowly but inexorably becoming almost completely paralyzed, requiring 24-hour nursing care. He lost his voice for good in 1985, and eventually a single muscle in his cheek attached to a sensor became the only way he could communicate with the outside world. Throughout, however, his powerful intellect was unimpaired, and he continued to work writing scientific publications and publishing 15 books. Many of these were for the general public, including five science-themed novels with his daughter, Lucy. In addition, he contributed to multiple film and TV productions on science and stated that he had no intention of retiring.

Hawking died at home on March 14, 2018 at age 76, outliving his prognosis by 53 years.

Hawking clearly had one of the long-lived variants of the ALS syndrome. Somehow, the death of motor neurons slowed, and the key neurons innervating his ability to breathe were relatively spared, all of this without significantly affecting his intellectual capabilities and remarkably not diminishing his will to keep on participating in life.

People from all walks of life and span of ages are devastated by ALS. Early onset, mostly genetic or inherited, forms strike younger adults, but most cases of ALS develop in middle age or later, ending many productive and high-impact careers. The disease is no respecter of success or contributions to society. Table 2.1 lists a few accomplished and well-known individuals who died with ALS. There are many more thousands who succumbed to the disease.

TODAY'S PUBLIC FACE OF ALS RESEARCH: THE ICE BUCKET CHALLENGE

ALS researchers have chronically struggled to fund their work. In midsummer 2014, a social media-driven fund-raising event unexpectedly changed the game.

Although some ALS research is being done in the pharmaceutical industry, as a rare disease with a relatively small number of individuals affected and with no clear path forward to therapeutics, it has generally received a low priority. The pharmaceutical industry has prioritized diseases with larger numbers of patients needing therapeutics. Funding by the National Institutes of Health (NIH) for academic institutions or small companies is spread among multiple diseases. Private foundations, such as the ALS Association and the Muscular Dystrophy Association, have been left to try to fill the gap in research funding for finding effective treatments for ALS.

Peter Frates, a Boston University alumnus and baseball player diagnosed with ALS in 2012, and Pat Quinn, diagnosed in 2013, were raising funds for ALS research. In July 2014, Quinn was posting on Facebook with friends about an ice bucket challenge, a popular way to raise funds for different causes in which people challenged others to videotape their coldwater dunking and to donate to charity. Frates picked this up and posted on Twitter. His message went viral in the Boston area.

The ease of use of social media, spirit of competition, and ease of entry combined to produce millions of Facebook postings and tweets. In August 2014, in the United States, Wikipedia viewings of the article on ALS went

Table 2.1   Notable People with ALS

Individual	Birth and Death Dates	Significance
Jason Becker	July 22, 1969–	American neoclassical metal guitarist and composer
Rob Borsellino	June 20, 1949–May 27, 2006	*Des Moines Register* newspaper columnist
Scott Brazil	May 12, 1955–April 17, 2006	Television producer and director of *Hill Street Blues* and other shows
Paul Celluchi	April 24, 1948–June 8, 2013	Former Massachusetts governor and U.S. ambassador to Canada
Ezzard Mack Charles	July 7, 1921–May 28, 1975	Boxer and former world heavyweight champion
Sid Collins	July 17, 1922–May 2, 1977	Radio voice of the Indianapolis 500 auto race
Dennis Day	May 21, 1916–June 22, 1988	Singer, comedian, and actor
Dieter Dengler	May 22, 1938–February 7, 2001	U.S. Navy pilot during the Vietnam War
Constantinos Doxiadis	May 14, 1913–June 28, 1975	Greek architect, urban planner, and visionary. Lead architect of Islamabad (Pakistan)
John Drury	January 4, 1927–November 25, 2007	Longtime ABC Chicago news anchor
Fokko du Cloux	December 20, 1954–November 10, 2006	Dutch mathematician and computer scientist
Jenifer Estess	February 17, 1963–December 16, 2003	Theater producer
Hal Finney	May 4, 1956–August 28, 2014	Bitcoin pioneer, first transaction
James Augustus "Catfish" Hunter	April 8, 1946–September 9, 1999	Baseball pitcher
Jon Imber	October 1, 1950–April 17, 2014	Renowned painter and Harvard professor of art
Jörg Immendorff	June 14, 1945–May 28, 2007	Controversial German painter and sculptor
Jacob Javits	May 18, 1904–March 7, 1986	New York politician

(*continued*)

Table 2.1   (continued)

Individual	Birth and Death Dates	Significance
Jimmie Johnstone	September 30, 1944–March 13, 2006	Scottish international football (soccer) star
Tony Judt	January 2, 1948–August 2, 2010	English American historian
Hans Keller	March 11, 1919–November 6, 1985	Austrian-born British musician and writer
Huddie William Ledbetter	January, 1888–December 6, 1949	Folk-blues musician
Charles Mingus	April 22, 1922–January 5, 1979	American jazz musician
Glenn Montgomery	March 31, 1967–June 28, 1998	NFL defensive tackle
David Niven	March 1, 1910–July 29, 1983	English actor, memoirist, and novelist
Richard Olney	December 15, 1947–January 27, 2012	Neurologist, ALS physician, and researcher
Sidney Osborn	May 17, 1884–May 25, 1948	Former four-term governor of Arizona
Mike Porcaro	May 29, 1955–March 15, 2015	American bass player
Mary Marr "Polly" Pratt	January 29, 1939–July 27, 2011	Film producer, production designer, and screenwriter
Diane Pretty	November 15, 1958–May 11, 2002	British right-to-die advocate
Franz Rosenzweig	December 25, 1886–December 10, 1929	Philosopher and religious thinker
Stanley Sadie	October 30, 1930–March 21, 2005	British musicologist, music critic, editor, and Commander of the Order of the British Empire
Ed Sadowski	January 19, 1931–November 6, 1993	American Baseball catcher and coach
Morrie Schwartz	December 20, 1916–November 4, 1995	Sociology professor at Brandeis University and author
Dmitri Shostakovich	September 25, 1903–August 9, 1975	Russian composer and pianist

(continued)

Table 2.1   (continued)

Individual	Birth and Death Dates	Significance
Lane Smith	April 29, 1936–June 13, 2005	American actor
Jon Stone	April 13, 1931–April 9, 1997	American writer, director, and producer, cocreator of *Sesame Street*
Maxwell D. Taylor	August 26, 1901–April 19, 1987	U.S. Army general, diplomat, and chairman of the Joint Chiefs of Staff
Orlando Thomas	October 21, 1972–November 9, 2014	NFL defensive safety
Ian Trethowan	October 20, 1922–December 12, 1990	Radio and TV journalist, director general of the BBC
Mao Tse-Tung	December 26, 1893–September 9, 1976	Chinese premier and author of the Great Cultural Revolution
Kevin Turner	June 12, 1969–March 24, 2016	New England Patriots football fullback
Roy Walford	June 29, 1924–April 27, 2004	Gerontologist, pioneer of the caloric restriction diet
Henry A. Wallace	October 7, 1888–November 18, 1965	33rd vice president of the United States
George Yardley III	November 3, 1928–August 12, 2004	First NBA player to score 2,000 points in a season
Michael Zaslow	November 1, 1942–December 6, 1998	American actor

NBA = National Basketball Association; NFL = National Football League.

from an average of 163,300 views a month to 2.89 million, and there were similar increases in the German and Spanish Wikipedia versions. In the United States as a result of the 2014 event, the ALS Association raised over $115 million from 2.5 million donors, and $220 million was raised globally. Donations have decreased since the initial ALS Ice Bucket Challenge spike, but using social media to engage the public to increase the visibility of the disease and the people suffering from it is now considered an effective fund-raising tool for the cause. They have been able to crowd source funding for scientists and physicians to jump-start finding effective therapies, in the hope of driving progress to a cure. Already three new genes linked to ALS have been discovered with funds from the ALS Ice Bucket Challenge.

Thanks to publicity phenomena such as the Ice Bucket Challenge, the plight of ALS patients moved out of the shadows into the public eye and generated enthusiasm (and funding) for progress against this disease. Recent scientific findings have also identified a number of features of ALS that are common to other neurodegenerative diseases, so ALS research and avenues for discovery of effective therapeutics will benefit from progress in those other areas.

This chapter described the recognition by clinicians of the different ways in which ALS can present and the confusion that caused for diagnosis, which lead to a search for causes and risk factors, despite the lack of effective presymptomatic diagnosis or predictive animal models. Early clinical trials produced only two medications that have, at best, a modest effect on the rate of functional decline and survival. We will next delve more deeply into what is known about possible causes of ALS and introduce the effects of risk factors that are not direct causes in their own right but that, in some cases, contribute to the development of ALS and the onset of symptoms.

3

Causes and Risk Factors

What causes ALS? Why, over 140 years after Charcot, do we not have the answer? In short, we don't really know what causes ALS because we do not know when the disease starts, only when its symptoms appear. The inciting events of ALS are possibly least understood of all of the neurodegenerative diseases. ALS announces itself to an individual by its symptoms—at first a barely noticeable weakened muscular response in a leg, foot, arm, or hand or a twitching of facial muscles. It is a disease that occurs later in life and for many patients comes as a complete surprise. By the time the symptoms and signs become obvious enough to be diagnosed as ALS, the disease process is well advanced. Investigators suspect that some individuals may begin life already with the disease process present, with others joining at later stages depending on their personal combination of genetic, environmental, and other factors. Knowing what to look for in biomarkers that present before the symptoms, the earlier the better, offers the best hope for successful intervention and a cure for ALS.

ALS lacks effective treatments with significant symptomatic relief or slowing of disease progression, much less a cure. What causes the loss of function of the motor neurons, the nerves that signal muscles to contract, is the subject of intense investigation. Cellular pathways are disrupted in a variety of ways. The problem is that a host of genetic and nongenetic risk factors also seem to impact motor neuron function in ALS, but none of them can be said to "cause" the disease on their own.

DETERMINING WHAT CAUSES ALS

Although it has been commonly assumed that the clinical onset of ALS disease (symptoms) occurs at the same time as or very shortly after the onset of the pathological disease process, this is not necessarily the case. In another, much more common neurodegenerative disorder, Alzheimer's disease, pathological changes occur silently for up to decades before the symptoms of this common neurodegenerative disease appear. Only by correlation with autopsy and recently developed brain imaging of pathology in living patients do we know that the Alzheimer's disease state is well established before cognitive impairment and memory loss are detectable. This may explain why therapeutic trials in symptomatic Alzheimer's disease have been disappointing.

Convincing evidence of symptomatically silent disease progression is currently lacking in human ALS. Even tests for motor neuron function and muscle abnormalities, biomarkers of neuromuscular function, fail to reliably predict the onset of symptoms the individual can feel. Absence of evidence, though, is not true evidence of absence. We can only conclude that we have not yet found the informative clues. The rare hereditary (familial) forms of ALS that show earlier and more consistent ages of onset have given investigators places to begin revealing pathways involved in disease progression. By expressing the mutant genes in model organisms, they can follow the consequences of each genetic change, as the organisms develop features of ALS looking for how different processes are affected.

Unfortunately, animal models of familial ALS where the genetic mutation is introduced do not faithfully reproduce human ALS, even human familial ALS, which they most closely resemble. However, they are useful for identifying alterations in biological processes that have also been found in humans. Many of the animal model changes have been seen in both fALS and ALS, and they have been observed in models as early as conception, during embryonic growth and development, and shortly after birth. Compensatory processes, which preserve function for at least some period of time, can also be observed.

When these protective mechanisms are eventually overcome either by further growth and development or by exposure to risk factors later in adult life, presymptomatic functional changes appear. They are soon followed by the clinical symptoms of impaired motor function and diagnosis of ALS. These observations suggest a disease model for ALS that encompasses the whole life span. By the time that clinical symptoms are evident, it is very likely that irreversible damage has occurred, and from this point, the rapid progression of the clinical part of the disease may be insurmountable. Early identification of incipient ALS individuals would likely improve the chances of successfully intervening therapeutically before symptomatic ALS diagnosis.

Hereditary Contributions

Many neurodegenerative diseases have genetic components that influence the probability of the disease. *Heritability* is observed as the occurrence of the disease in offspring across multiple generations. In the most common neurodegenerative diseases, such as Alzheimer's and Parkinson's diseases, a small number of genes exist that when changes (mutations) are present in their DNA sequence in an individual, with very high probability the changes result in disease. The disease often has an earlier age of onset, but a similar progression rate, and symptom severity pattern. Each individual carries two copies of each gene, one from each of the parents. When one inherited mutated copy of the gene is enough to cause a defect or disease, this mode of inheritance is called *dominant*. There can be different genes or different mutations that require two copies of the mutated gene, one from each of the parents, to cause the disease. These genes are termed *recessive*, and they can appear to skip generations when two active copies of these genes are not present.

Gene mutations rarely account for more than a small percentage of all cases of most neurodegenerative diseases, and ALS is no exception, in that only about 10 percent of ALS cases can be assigned as dominantly inherited. The first dominant ALS gene mutation to be described was identified in 1993 as SOD1, superoxide dismutase-1, an enzyme whose activity was to break down toxic free-radical chemicals in the cell. Oddly, very few of the over 150 mutations scattered throughout the SOD1 protein affect its enzymatic activity. This lack of effect of mutations on the enzyme's activity and their effects when present at different positions all over the protein indicated that the whole SOD1 molecule was involved. The result of the disease mutations was that SOD1 misfolded easily and accumulated in clumps in motor neurons, which then lost their connections to target muscles. SOD1 is only one of the genes strongly genetically connected to ALS. In 60–80 percent of patients with inherited (familial) ALS, the most common mutations are in C9orf72 (40 percent), SOD1 (20 percent), FUS (1–5 percent), and TARBDP = TDP43 (1–5 percent).

In addition to these classical genetic (hereditary) strong influences on ALS, other genetic influences arise from varying weak contributions of combinations of myriad different genes out of the 19,000 that code for proteins thought to be in the human genome. Individually these genes do not have a discernible effect on the probability of developing ALS, but different groupings of mutations or variations in these genes can generate an overall effect—a risk factor.

Multiple Forms of ALS

The multiple forms of ALS briefly described in chapter 1 differ primarily in the initial localization of the loss of muscular function and the rates of progression of functional deficits. It is not clear at this time what governs where and when the disease symptoms will appear first. As the multiple genetic and environmental contributors are better defined and their impact determined, it may be possible to apply the concepts and technology of precision medicine to analyze the many possibilities and thereby provide insight to specifically address the different manifestations of ALS.

Cognitive Involvement

Charcot's description of ALS from what he knew at the time restricted the symptoms to nerve-muscle connection with sparing of sensory and mental functions. The existence of variants with definable characteristics related to motor neuron dysfunction and muscle denervation was recognized, especially those connected to longer or shorter survival time or those that responded to different management strategies. By 2000, improved clinical diagnostic procedures were identifying cognitive symptoms in a subpopulation of ALS patients, comprising 20–50 percent of diagnosed ALS cases. The nature of most of these cognitive deficits closely resembled those of another neurodegenerative disease: frontotemporal dementia.

The mental functions and the brain regions affected in FTD are distinct from those of Alzheimer's disease, the most common dementing disease. Autopsy revealed that in addition to motor neuron pathology affecting muscles, deposits of the TDP43 protein were found in these ALS patients in the brain areas serving cognitive function, where TDP43 deposits were found in frontotemporal dementia patients. In classic FTD, muscle function is not affected. It appeared that the pathologies in brain areas containing degenerating motor cortical neurons and the TDP43 deposit-bearing nonmotor cortical neurons were converging in the brains of ALS-FTD patients but were not identical. It is currently unknown why only some ALS patients develop TDP43 pathology and only some cognitive and behavioral symptoms.

In hindsight, this overlap of pathologies should not have been surprising. Although ALS is conceived of as a strictly motor neuron and muscle disease, in the more prevalent neurodegenerative diseases not affecting muscle function, it is common for mixed pathologies of different diseases to be found upon autopsy in the same individual. Sometimes patients show symptoms of both diseases. Common features in the biochemical mechanisms that lead to propagation of the protein clumping in neurons in all of these diseases may be responsible for enhancing the probability of the different pathologies.

Regional Spread of Neuron Death in ALS

Both the nerve damage and the loss of muscle function in ALS start focally, initially affecting a small number of the muscle fibers that comprise a muscle, weakening its strength of contraction until eventually the nervous input is silenced. Without that input, the muscle will not respond and begins to break down (atrophy). The neuronal dysfunction and muscle atrophy spread throughout the affected limb. Autopsy studies reveal that the dysfunction is coincident with the wasting of affected motor neuronal processes and with the accumulation of *inclusion bodies,* clumps of cellular debris inside the nerve processes that are the hallmark of ALS.

The same process is occurring in the motor cortex, the part of the brain that controls voluntary muscle activity. For unknown reasons, in classical ALS only motor neurons are affected by these processes. Sensory nerves physically right next to motor neurons in the spinal cord look normal, and sensory functions are unaffected. Some ALS researchers have suggested that the dysfunction is being transmitted between connected nerve cells, leading to the concept that "cells that are wired together die together."

This spread of pathology and loss of function is also common to other neurodegenerative diseases, such as Alzheimer's, Parkinson's, and frontotemporal dementia. Although these other diseases affect only the brain, not muscles, the spread of neuronal mayhem is analogous. The brain regions that are connected by neurons, which are different in these diseases characteristic of the symptoms of the individual diseases. Preventing this spread of dysfunction through neuronal connections could be an effective therapeutic approach for multiple diseases.

WHY DO ONLY MOTOR NEURONS DIE?

A visible pathology is evident in ALS patients at autopsy. Motor neurons serving the muscle groups that weaken and degenerate during the symptomatic disease phase are disconnected from the muscles, and muscle mass decreases dramatically. Like many types of neurons, once motor neurons degenerate, they not replaced. The pathology begins focally, often in the motor cortex, and spreads among connected neuronal pathways. The identity of the initial cause of the neuronal degeneration is unknown and may differ somewhat between individuals, depending on their genetic composition and exposure to risk factors.

There may also be influences fed back from the muscles that the neurons control. The energy-generating stations of the neurons, their mitochondria, are damaged, producing toxic free-radical chemical reactions that overwhelm cellular protective mechanisms, and regulation of the rate of motor neuron signaling to voluntary muscles fails. The motor neurons become hypersensitive to input and overactive, causing further damage to the neuron and the loss of a type of neuron that normally manages the activity of the motor neuron.

Surprisingly, despite the general chaos, during most of the disease process, only the motor neurons connected to voluntary muscles are obviously severely affected. Other neuronal types, such as sensory neurons, and certain motor neurons, such as those controlling eye movement and sphincter closure, unexplainably remain unaffected, at least until very late in the disease.

Misfolding Proteins

The current main hypothesis for the driver of motor neuron degeneration in ALS is the accumulation of the very noticeable protein clumps called *inclusions*. They are formed from proteins that fail to fold to their normal functional structure and instead accumulate in inactive or toxic clumps. Support for this derives from studies on fALS in animal models, in which the human mutations of genes linked to ALS are introduced into their genetic material. Mutations in four genes coding for the C9orf72, SOD1, FUS, and TDP43 proteins account for 60–80 percent of all fALS cases. In most subtypes of nonfamilial ALS, normal TDP43 is the main protein that accumulates, although in this case, for some reason it is not due to a mutation in TDP43.

All of these proteins have an inherent tendency to misfold, lose their normal function, and form abnormal structures, which accumulate and impair normal protein processing and turnover in the cell. The inability to adequately break down damaged or no-longer-needed proteins leads to protein accumulation, which is disruptive to cell function. Formation of the protein aggregates disturbs a variety of vital cellular control networks. They impair mitochondrial energy production and also disrupt critical communication with and inside the nucleus. These aggregates clog multiple different transport pathways within the neuron, including the traffic in the axon, the long cell process that extends from the cell body to the synapses that target muscle fibers.

Nucleic Acid Dysfunction

C9orf72, FUS, and TDP43 proteins are all involved in the control of the processing of the ribonucleic acid (RNA) intermediates produced from the deoxyribonucleic acid (DNA) of the active genes in the genome. They normally bind RNA in the nucleus and translocate it to the cytoplasm, the fluid that fills the inside of the cell. By binding the RNA, they protect it from degradation and control further processing. In neurons, these protein-RNA complexes are often transported to distant sites in the cell. Mutations in these proteins disrupt the nucleus-cytoplasm transport and lead to clumping of these protein-RNA complexes, which disrupts their function. These same mutations cause fALS. Proteins, such as NEK1 and C21orf2, are involved in DNA repair, variants of which can cause ALS. How they achieve their effects remains to be established.

Excitotoxicity

Neurons have an optimal rate of activity. Too much or too little and they will die. Overly active neurons suffer from excitotoxicity. In ALS, the upper motor neurons make connections with lower motor neurons in the spinal cord and regulate their activity. Lower motor neurons in the spinal column use acetylcholine as a neurotransmitter in order to control the muscles that they directly contact. The upper motor neurons are particularly sensitive to toxicity, due to overstimulation by the neurotransmitter, they respond to, a chemical called glutamate. They have more of a receptor that very strongly responds to normal levels of glutamate, flooding the upper motor neurons with toxic concentrations of calcium ion. Making things worse, in ALS patients the surrounding astroglial cells, responsible for mopping up excess glutamate neurotransmitter, are impaired in glutamate uptake for an unknown reason. Riluzole (Rilutek), the FDA-approved therapeutic for ALS, reduces the amount of glutamate that is released by the upper motor neurons, which would be expected to directly have a protective effect on upper motor neurons. This would have an indirect effect on lower motor neurons, but it is unclear how much of the therapeutic effect of riluzole is due to this drug-action mechanism.

Other Contributors

While major pathologic drivers of ALS are quite characteristic of chronic neurodegenerative disease, in ALS, a number of other processes are affected that more generally impact overall nervous system function at some stage. They are not specific to motor neurons and are not the primary instigators of ALS. Their impact can be at any disease stage, from priming motor neurons and muscles to contributing instigating factors that drive disease progression. The only therapeutics available for ALS broadly address these contributing factors without selectively targeting any one of them.

Cellular Environment

Nonneuronal cells in the vicinity of the motor neurons under attack also respond to clues from the dysfunctional neurons generating a hostile environment. The main players about which the most is known are *astroglia*, *oligodendroglia*, and *microglia*. All provide support of some kind for the health and functionality of the neurons that they contact. Astroglia provide a variety of protein factors important for neuronal function and scavenge excess neurotransmitter to prevent neuronal overexcitation. Oligodendroglia, cells that enwrap the neuronal axons with a lipid-protein myelin sheath, provide electrical insulation as well as physical structural organization and secrete a variety of protein-supporting factors for the motor neurons. Microglia are the brain's version of macrophages. These are mobile white blood cells that in the nervous system defend against infections, scavenge and dispose of debris, prune nonfunctional synapses, and provide a variety of protein factors to induce cellular protective responses against insults of various types.

Under normal conditions, these glial cell types cooperate to ensure proper neuronal function and to protect against infection and overactive immune-system responses. Under pathological conditions, their responses lose their coordination and, in some cases, even conflict, and the neurons are the losers. The pathological conditions in some individuals can be from the effects of the expression in one or more of the glial types of familial ALS genes or even gene variants statistically associated with ALS but without a dominant effect. They can also be simply responding to how the other cells, including neurons, are reacting to what is happening in their environment.

Oxidative Stress

Oxidative stress is a condition caused by the abnormal exposure of a set of normally sequestered chemical reactions in cells that modify the molecular structures of important components in ways that prevent them from functioning properly. These modifications can alter the structure and destroy the functions of some proteins, while their attack on lipid membrane components alters cell-membrane integrity, causing leakiness and abnormal cell function. A normal cell is able to organize and restrict access to the systems it uses to perform the chemistry required to generate energy, to synthesize molecules needed for cellular functions, and to detoxify potentially dangerous molecules in its environment.

The mitochondrion, an organelle inside cells, contains a number of systems that employ a series of chemical reactions to produce the energy that cells need. Mitochondrial dysfunction caused by mutant SOD1 and TDP43 impairs mitochondrial energy production and breaks down the protective barriers, which exposes the cell to free radicals leaking from the damaged mitochondria inside them. The free-radical scavenging of dietary vitamin E is likely responsible for its effects on reducing risk for ALS. Neutralizing free radicals may also be part of the therapeutic effect of edaravone (Radicava) in treating diagnosed ALS.

Neuroinflammation

Neuroinflammation is the complex biological response of the nervous system to harmful stimuli. An important component of the neurotoxic environment in ALS is due to the microglial cells in the vicinity of the motor neurons. They respond to the affected motor neurons by the release of protein factors; some are supportive of neuronal function, but others further stress the injured neurons. These factors also impact other glial types, which contribute their own responses. Determining which of the factors and the different cell types in this complex web of interactions are responsible for the progression of ALS and onset of symptoms remains highly challenging. Achieving therapeutic selectivity by differentially modulating factor production or the factor effect will be more difficult. Available anti-inflammatory drugs are generally not selective for individual factors.

Viruses

Infections of HIV and poliovirus can cause motor neuron dysfunction and muscle paralysis, but these are not ALS. Currently, there is no evidence that ALS is directly caused by viral infections. However, there are suggestions that retroviruses like HIV may contribute in a noninfectious way to a number of diseases and ALS in particular. Our genome contains a large amount of residual DNA from retroviral infections that occurred in very distant ancestors, was incorporated into the human germ line, and was passed along from generation to generation. Originally considered "junk DNA" because it had no discernable function, sequencing revealed that around 8 percent of the DNA in our genome consists of inactive retroviral genes, most of which are defective, due to a buildup of mutations over generations.

Reactivation of some of these retroviral genes or fragments of them can lead to production of a protein or peptide with a biological activity. Expression of the human endogenous retrovirus K (HERV-K) genome has been detected in a subgroup of patients with ALS but not in healthy controls. One of the three genes in the HERV-K genome codes for expression of a protein that is selectively toxic to motor neurons when tested in mouse models. It is also suspected to be involved in multiple sclerosis. Interestingly, expression from the HERV-K genome is activated by the TDP43 protein, a key player in familial ALS and in ALS-FTD. The potential for inherited HERV-K gene reactivation by TDP43 has sparked antiretroviral therapy clinical trials to suppress HERV-K in ALS patients. Reactivation of dormant retroviral genes could potentially be triggered by environmental exposures and be specific to tissue, cell, development, or maturational stage.

RISK FACTORS

ALS seems to occur naturally only in humans. Determining how the disease begins and progresses depends heavily on work done with cellular and animal models that have been genetically modified to produce the genetic mutants identified in human patients with fALS. Causes of sporadic ALS, which accounts for 90 percent of ALS cases, are much more uncertain. It appears that there are a variety of stressors that, alone or in combination, can achieve the dysregulation of voluntary motor neuron function acting at different points during the long, preclinical period of ALS that finally causes affected cells to "fall off the cliff" and degenerate. It is not understood how these risk factors differentially impact individuals, but this is important in developing early stage interventions to slow or block disease progression.

ALS shares a complex multifactorial nature with many other neurodegenerative diseases. Variable susceptibility of individuals and a spectrum of ages of onset and rates of progression initially hampered definition of ALS until Charcot described the archetype symptoms and named the disease. We now understand that this variability is an indication of the interplay of multiple factors that can impact individuals differently. Parsing out the individual contributions and their effect on the individual's susceptibility and clinical expectations will be difficult, although defining categories may be useful, particularly if there are differential responses to treatments.

Genetic Contributions to ALS

The proportion of the risk of ALS that is determined by heritability has been estimated by studying twins. About 60 percent of the risk is determined by heritability—due to some of the estimated 19,000 protein-coding genes in an individual's genetic code and its regulation. More than 30 of those genes that code for proteins have been connected to a major risk for ALS. The remaining 40 percent is determined by the interaction of genetic components with nongenetic contributions from environmental factors, occupational exposures, and lifestyle exposures. The influence of nongenetic components in the absence of the genetic components is thought not to be of sufficient magnitude to cause disease, but the cumulative effect over time on genetic contribution eventually crosses a threshold. Once started, the degenerative process is self-sustaining and irreversible.

Familial ALS versus Sporadic ALS

In fALS patients, who constitute about 10 percent of all cases of ALS, 60–80 percent have a mutation in a single gene that strongly drives the disease in that individual. The most common genes (percent of fALS cases) with this large effect are C9orf72 (40 percent), SOD1 (20 percent), FUS (1–5 percent), and TARBDP = TDP43 (1–5 percent). A rare fALS mutation on the X-chromosome in the UBQLN2 gene coding for the ubiquilin-2 protein is dominantly expressed. Because it is on the X-chromosome, it is not passed from males in one generation to males in the next generation.

By contrast, in sporadic ALS the individual genetic risk factors are likely to be rare (0.1–5.0 percent) gene forms of a number of genes, each with intermediate-to-large effects (oligogenic). This situation is distinct from a number of other disease conditions, such as neuropsychiatric disorders (e. g., schizophrenia), in which there are a large number of genetic variants, each with small effects that add together to cause disease (polygenic).

Blurring the distinction between fALS and sporadic ALS, an increasing number of genetic studies show multiple overlapping of sets of genes involved in the two forms. This suggests that the division of ALS into familial and sporadic disease types is an oversimplification. Except for the earlier age of onset and often more rapid progression rate of fALS, the symptoms and pathology of the two forms are highly similar, although not identical. An international whole-genome sequencing project initiated by Project MinE is sequencing the complete genomes of 15,000 ALS cases and 7,500 controls (non-ALS). The study is intended to better define the contributions of individual genes and genome structures to the risk of ALS.

Epigenetics and ALS

Epigenetics, literally "on top of genetics," is a term whose current use was defined in 2008. It refers to regulation of how the genetic code of the DNA containing the blueprint for an organism is used. The DNA code is like a computer hard drive containing information, and epigenetics is like the software that controls how the information on the hard drive is used by telling it what to do. Epigenetics can also be thought of as punctuation that specifies which of the DNA sentence words are to be read, how, and when. A special *marking* mechanism provides an extra layer of control that modulates which genes are expressed and which are repressed.

The DNA code for the gene itself remains unchanged. What is being controlled is only when it is being used and how much. A way for an individual organism to reversibly adapt its responses to its experiences, epigenetics is a point at which environmental effects and exposure to toxic (heavy metals, poisons) or protective conditions (exercise and healthy diet) can control gene expression. Even experiences like the amount of sleep an individual gets, chronic stress, prolonged malnutrition, or starvation have an impact. This marking mechanism is how experience can influence disease and health without changing the basic genetic code itself.

Although in mammals most of the epigenetic marks are removed from the DNA when gametes are produced and during fertilization to reset control for the embryo, some marks can be retained. Thus, some epigenetic control is itself heritable, causing some genes to be silenced or activated across generations. An example of transgenerational epigenetic inheritance would be observed changes in metabolism due to events such as extreme starvation experienced during the Irish Potato Famine (1845–1849) in a grandparent generation that linger in the next and even later generations.

The apparent epigenetic contribution to ALS further muddles determining the genetic component's contribution to ALS. The current understanding of epigenetic mechanisms is far from complete, which also makes deciphering the processes driving ALS much more difficult. Overlap in the functions of the products of multiple genes implicated in contributing to disease also hampers design of potential therapies.

Genes Connected with ALS

Many human noninfectious diseases are monogenic; their cause is due to mutations in a single gene. Online Mendelian Inheritance in Man, an online database of human genes and genetic disorders, lists thousands of these diseases. They are rare, much less common than ALS, and they are not strongly associated with risk factors in addition to the mutant gene. ALS is complicated by having disease processes driven in some individuals by single genes and by multiple genes in other individuals. In addition, a strong effect of gene-regulation mechanisms sensitive to environment, occupation, and lifestyle in the broadest sense increase the risk of ALS.

Monogenic versus Multigenic

Family-based studies are used to discover variants in genes associated with disease. Slight changes in the structure of the protein the gene codes for, or how much or how little the gene produces of its product, can cause physiological alterations that lead to disease. When there is a family history of a disease, those gene changes are observed in subsequent generations, an indication of an inherited characteristic. When these single gene effects are large and no other gene changes are involved, the type of disease is described as *monogenic* and *familial*. There are a small number of these large-effect genes (C9orf72, SOD1, FUS, and TARBDP = TDP43).

Where it gets complicated is when rare changes in a number of other genes happen to be all present at the same time, which is called *multigenic* disease. None of the individual changes in those genes on their own will cause disease, but the effect of their sum total is enough to tip the health-disease balance. If those particular genes are any of the genes whose functions converge on the same cellular processes, the variable presence of gene variants in families among individuals can combine in ways that make the occurrence of ALS appear sporadic or to skip one or more generations.

Epigenetic Regulation

Because the contribution of multiple gene variants to the disrupted physiology in ALS can be influenced by the relative activities of those genes, epigenetic mechanisms that control that activity can also govern the risk of ALS. *Epigenetic regulation* is likely a major mechanism by which seemingly nongenetic processes can control disease incidence. New technologies are now being used to learn the molecular mechanisms underlying epigenetic controls in order to harmonize the disease-causing factors and to provide an avenue for possible therapeutic intervention.

Epigenetic regulation can cause changes at any stage of life, with the effects evident only later in life. Beginning in utero, the fetus is subject to maternal influences, hormonal and otherwise, that can impose epigenetic regulation on genes. This regulation can have lasting effects that influence growth and development of the fetus, the newborn, and the growing child.

Demographics

Demographics are a description of a population in the form of statistics of the characteristics of the individuals in that population. The characteristics chosen for each study depend on the intended use of the information. Typically they include age, gender, education and income level, marital status, occupation, race, ethnicity, and often other characteristics such as religion as well as birth and death rates. Population statistics are an overall summary that loses the individual characteristics. On the other hand, by smoothing out individual differences, overall trends associated with groups of people, if large enough in magnitude, can inform on risk factors that would evade a standard genetic analysis of genome data. Such studies can be useful in assessing the contribution of environmental, occupational, and lifestyle factors to the incidence of ALS.

Ethnicity and Race

These two terms tend to be confused in common usage. *Ethnicity* has to do with sociological factors (culture), while *race* refers to biological factors like genetics. Overall incidence of ALS differs by geographic location, which combines both race (genetics) and ethnicity (cultural/economic) influences. For example, the overall incidence of ALS from a survey through 2015 of the literature over 42 locations in 11 subcontinental regions was 1.68 ALS cases per 100,000 people. Males have a higher incidence than females. Within that survey, in Northern Europe the incidence was 1.89; in East Asia (China and Japan), it was 0.83, and in South Asia (Iran), it was 0.73. In Europe, North America, and New Zealand, the incidence of ALS was 1.81. Overall in the United States a different study over 2009–2011 (by a European group), non-Hispanic incidence of ALS was 1.65, while Hispanic incidence was 0.57. While the individual numbers vary between studies, the differences remain relatively constant. From the data analyzed, it is not possible to exclude the contributions of ancestral origin from environmental or lifestyle influences. These geographical regions also contain variable heterogeneity in the racial content of their populations.

Differences in ALS incidence also exist between races. In the same United States study, in data from 2009–2011, the overall (combined all races) incidence was 1.44 per 100,000 people. Whites suffer a higher incidence (1.79) than Blacks (0.8) or Asians (0.76). These incidence rates by race did not significantly depend on income, poverty, home ownership, or gender. Thus, biological effects with a genetic basis are likely responsible for driving the differences. As in the study of ethnicity, confounding factors prevent analyzing the data to determine the influence of environmental or lifestyle factors.

Nongenetic Contributions

When searching for causes of illnesses, researchers try to identify common experiences of individuals showing characteristic disease symptoms.

In the case of a sudden epidemic of intestinal ailments, was it drinking from a common water source or eating certain foods? Correlation of experiences with the presence of disease is also helpful for conditions for which there is no single proven cause or strong genetic connection. While not the cause, per se, these associations can provide valuable clues to the combinations of insults, events that can cause the disease to start or progress.

For ALS, the correlation of life experiences with increased incidence and prevalence of the disease is divided into four broad categories. None is capable of causing ALS on its own, nor is it certain that exposure to all of them will result in ALS. The probability of ALS increases with exposure to multiple factors, and it is not clear which factors have the most impact, as they often vary among different populations. Clusters of higher incidence of ALS in populations suggest that those people are exposed to shared environmental risk factors. There is no single gene variant or environmental risk factor that can be conclusively linked to the onset of sporadic ALS.

When considering experiences of an individual as risk factors for ALS, it is important to remember that the individual magnitudes of their effect are relatively small and may or may not be additive. The impact of the effect depends on when it occurred during the individual's lifetime and for how long the experience lasted. Since risk factor calculations are a statistical measure, an adequate number of people have to be included for meaningful results, especially for a relatively uncommon disease like ALS. Many studies simply do not have enough participants to reach a solid statistically valid conclusion.

Combination of the results of multiple studies into a meta-analysis is one way to provide improved data analysis, but it comes with a loss of control of variables. Only factors with a large-enough effect to be distinguishable from the background can be detected. Nongenetic contributions generally increase the risk less than twofold, with at most a few times the average incidence. These influences are much less than genetic factors that are considered causative. However, the nongenetic effects are taken as support for a multistage ALS disease process, where different factors have effects at certain stages of the disease and not at others, so the magnitude of effect depends on when an exposure occurs. This multistage mechanism will be explained in chapter 4.

The effect of risk factors is most often considered for the onset of disease symptoms, but they can also have an effect on the speed at which the full expression of ALS symptoms develops. A measure of the progression rate of the disease is defined as the time between first symptoms and diagnosis. Progression rate is usually inversely associated with survival time; the longer the time between first symptoms and sufficient progression to permit diagnosis, the longer the survival time after diagnosis.

Environment

Exposure to pesticides and certain organic solvents, particularly certain agricultural chemicals, is linked to increased risk for developing ALS. When the pesticides cis-chlordane and pentachlorobenzene, persistent in the environment, are at levels detectable in the blood, this is strongly linked to increased risk. Engagement in agriculture or living in a rural setting are not in themselves risks for ALS, as long as blood levels of pesticides and certain agricultural chemicals are low. Environmental levels of heavy metals, such as lead and mercury, are inconsistently linked to ALS. There is weak evidence that exposure to electromagnetic fields, such as those surrounding high voltage electrical transmission lines, or high-intensity radar is connected with ALS. Electric shock can cause a neuromuscular defect, but the lack of progression of muscle degeneration does not support it as a risk factor for ALS.

Occupation

Military service, particularly in the U.S. armed forces and less so in the French, Italian, or British military, is linked to an increased incidence of ALS. The effect is dependent on whether the individuals were deployed in active service and whether their service occurred before 1950. Exactly what in the deployed experience contributes to the increased incidence is not clear. Injury, explosions and their related chemical exposure, especially to Agent Orange in Vietnam, heavy metals, and solvents along with high levels of stress are all part of the deployed military experience and are associated with increased risk for ALS. Employment in construction, manufacturing, mechanical, or painting occupations is also associated with increased risk for ALS, most likely due to exposure to cleaning chemicals and other solvents.

Lifestyle

Smoking seems to have little effect on ALS incidence, but when comparing people who have never smoked to those who have smoked during their life, it is clear that there is a significant adverse effect on survival time once diagnosed with ALS. This effect is especially prominent in women. Smoking after diagnosis is linked to shorter survival.

A low body mass index (BMI) is a consistent risk factor for ALS. A BMI greater or equal to 25 at any age lowers the risk of ALS. Overweight or obese individuals are at lower risk for ALS, but they may suffer from other disorders linked to their weight.

Mechanisms of ALS may be influenced by diet, particularly those factors that impact oxidative stress, mitochondrial dysfunction, and inflammation in neurons, including the motor neurons affected in ALS. Consumption of vitamin E, an antioxidant that reduces oxidative stress and improves mitochondrial function, reduces the risk of ALS, but vitamin E supplements have no effect on the progression of ALS or survival time once diagnosed. Consumption of different types of fat and cholesterol minimally affects the incidence of ALS or survival. Malnutrition negatively impacts survival. Severe vitamin D deficiency accelerates the rate of decline by fourfold, drastically shortening life expectancy.

High Physical Activity

Physical activity and fitness are commonly considered healthy for the general population. Many diseases and conditions are improved by exercise. For most people experiencing moderate amounts of physical activity, using muscles helps keep them and their nerve connections healthy. However, for reasons not well understood, intense physical activity like organized or professional sports and a fit, lean athletic body (low BMI) increases the risk for ALS, while a higher BMI is protective. There is a reason that ALS is overrepresented among professional athletes. Lou Gehrig was a strong, fit individual. The ALS risk is higher in contact sports, suggesting that repetitive muscle and nerve trauma experienced may play a role in this enhancement.

Genetic and nongenetic risk factors on motor neuron function and survival play critical but not yet fully understood roles in modulating the cellular pathways of motor neurons in the presymptomatic stages of ALS. We will next focus on the signs that clinicians use to try to detect ALS before the patient experiences symptoms and the importance of the patient noticing those telltale symptoms.

4

Signs and Symptoms

Many diseases have *biomarkers*, defined as objective, quantifiable physical features or molecules that are associated with a particular disease state. Importantly, certain biomarkers can be used as a sign to detect the presence or stage of a disease state before the patient experiences symptoms, something they can feel or see. Familiar examples of signs are cholesterol levels or glucose levels in the blood, which are used as indicators of cardiovascular health and the presence or potential for diabetes, respectively. ALS currently lacks this type of biomarker to detect presymptomatic, early stage disease.

Meanwhile, ALS is currently diagnosed by its symptoms. In some cases, tests of electrophysiological measurements of muscle function can provide an early indication of impending onset of the disease's symptomatic phase. A diagnosis is arrived at after excluding a number of look-alike motor-function diseases with different prognoses for function and longevity. The diagnostic process for ALS will be described in more detail in chapter 5.

Current thinking about how ALS progresses undetected for most of its course is that progressing to the symptomatic stage involves multiple steps, each affected by different factors. This accounts for the complexity of risk factors impacting ALS and helps to explain the difficulties the disease presents for diagnosis and disease-modifying intervention. It makes it immediately apparent why shrinking the delay between symptom detection and clinical diagnosis is critical for the most effective management of functional decline. Indeed, the multistep disease model has been changing the way that cancer is thought about and treated. It has been useful in addressing a number of cancers allowing researchers to successfully systemize therapeutic approaches to this complex multifactorial disease.

ALS very likely does not suddenly begin when symptoms appear. An age-dependent disease consisting of *presymptomatic, symptom onset*, and *functional decline* phases, it is now believed to begin with a lengthy, symptomatically silent phase. During this initiating phase, predisposing factors like genetic makeup (inherited, epigenetic) and a variety of risk factors (random mutation, environmental exposures, smoking, military deployment, diet) impact processes in the vulnerable motor neurons and affected muscles. The time period over which these factors act could extend as far back as conception and could include development in the maternal environment, followed by growth and development into adulthood.

This multistep process is believed to describe the symptom-silent progression stage, with each step a result of multiple alternative pathways. Although this sounds like a hopeless muddle, analysis of incidence rates of first symptoms for different ages suggests that there are six steps, six *hits*, in the disease process leading to symptoms. Because there are multiple different ways that the same final state can be caused, such as with hits occurring in different orders but converging on similar mechanisms, ALS can be thought of as a syndrome.

While it doesn't specify a particular stepwise order, future identification of these steps could lead to the identification of valuable presymptomatic biomarkers for very early ALS processes. It also would provide for a personalized-medicine approach, in which interventions could be developed that would differ among subgroups of patients in the way that they impact disease progression to the symptomatic stage. An analogous multistage process likely describes the steps of functional decline after diagnosis, which has thus far proven resistant to therapeutic management.

THE IMPORTANCE OF NOTICING SYMPTOMS

Muscle weakness that begins focally and then painlessly spreads to nearby areas over succeeding weeks or months is often the first symptom that patients notice. Frequently the change is so minor that it is ignored at first, and primary care physicians may not pick up on the clue. The weakness can manifest simply as a delayed or lack of response to the intent to move a leg, arm, or the jaw. Another symptom is maintenance of a spontaneous reflex of the otherwise-weakened voluntary response of a limb to external stimulation. By the time a neurologist specializing in ALS sees the patient, often after a series of inconclusive evaluations, a year or more may have passed, during which the classical spread of ALS becomes well established. Often some respiratory dysfunction can already be detected. Special diagnostic testing is necessary to exclude ALS mimics, especially treatable disorders that share some features of ALS but require a different treatment and have different prognoses.

FAMILY TENDENCIES

Currently, functional symptoms are the earliest noticeable indication that the potential for ALS disease exists in an individual. Exceptions are in cases of familial forms of ALS, in which other family members suffered ALS due to a mutation in one of the major ALS risk-factor genes. These potent predisposing factors for ALS call for an aggressive approach to investigate suspicious symptoms quickly. Family members are also more likely to share the combination of gene variants inherited from their parents that may influence the probability of developing ALS. These gene variants do not have the ability to cause ALS on their own, unlike the familial risk-factor genes, but different combinations of these variants may increase the risk of developing ALS.

Coupled with the various genetic predisposing factors are risk factors frequently shared by family members, such as occupations with exposure to chemicals and environmental toxins like those in agriculture, mining, and military deployment. Combinations of the genetic variants may sensitize individuals to effects of environmental factors. While association of environmental factors with the risk for initiating and developing ALS is not consistent, previous exposure to some factors may affect the later development of the disease and the rate of functional decline of ALS after it is diagnosed.

TIME COURSE OF ALS PROGRESSION: SUBTYPES OF ALS

The impact of the delay between symptoms and before diagnosis depends on what type of ALS the patient has. Because the disease affects only certain muscle groups and not others, these groups are in different physical locations in the body, and since each of the groups are affected with different time courses or ages of onset, they can appear to be different diseases. At symptom onset, it is difficult to discern in individual patients which course the disease will take. These differences in presentation and the lack of predictive biomarkers make it difficult and time-consuming to accurately diagnose ALS. In addition, different diseases arising from other causes affect motor neuron function, causing similar symptoms that are not ALS. ALS mimics are important to distinguish because some of them are treatable and/or affect prognosis, including extended survival times. It is vital to get the diagnosis correct and to identify patients with the generally faster-progressing ALS spectrum of disorders in order to properly manage their care and symptoms.

Initially, painless weakness that progressively affects connected muscle groups is the neurologist's clue to ALS. Later, loss of motor neuron control causes pain from muscle cramping, and spasticity sets in. The most common form of the disease, accounting for about 70 percent of all cases, is termed *classical ALS*. Two-thirds of these cases initially affect the lower motor neurons in the spine, which control movement of the arms and legs. In the remaining one-third of cases, the function of upper motor neurons originating in the motor cortex region of the brain and controlling the face and neck are affected. Patients with this *bulbar* form often initially present with speech difficulties, which eventually evolve into difficulties in swallowing from the loss of control and wasting of facial muscles. Each of these major forms of classical ALS can be separated into subgroups depending on the details of the extent and regions affected as well as the order of development of symptoms. Spinal nerve dysfunction characterizes *flail arm, flail leg, hemiplegic,* and *pseudopolyneuritic* forms of ALS.

The second major form, encompassing 5–15 percent of cases of ALS, is a more recently recognized subtype that includes cognitive or behavioral changes, or both, along with either spinal or bulbar onset. *ALS-FTD* characteristically involves the combined pathologies of both ALS and frontotemporal dementia, which normally affect different brain regions that control different functions. In ALS-FTD, dementia results from the pathology in the frontotemporal brain region. In some cases, the dementia can present before the ALS muscle symptoms appear. Since both of the pure forms of the ALS and FTD diseases involve the misfolding of the TDP43 protein yet affect different brain modalities (muscle and cognition/behavior), it is not surprising that if conditions favoring misfolding of TDP43 protein exist in the brain that the symptoms of the two diseases can be coexpressed. About 40 percent of FTD patients have mild motor-neuron dysfunction, and a smaller proportion of those with the behavioral variant will develop ALS.

About 5 percent of ALS cases, mostly females, involve only the bulbar region, controlling muscles that power swallowing and speaking. *Pseudobulbar palsy* and *isolated bulbar palsy* differ from classical ALS cases in that they do not spread further and patients survive for years.

Other forms of ALS, accounting for 10 percent of ALS cases, also feature extended survival times. *Progressive spinal muscular atrophy* involves lower motor neuron dysfunction that remains localized for an extended period of time although it eventually progresses to respiratory failure. *Primary lateral sclerosis* involves only upper motor neurons where symptoms spread from bulbar to limbs. Survival in this form ranges from more than 10 years to normal life expectancy.

STAGES OF ALS: SYMPTOM APPEARANCE

Early in the progression of ALS, it can be difficult to recognize what is happening, much less suspect a diagnosis of this relatively unfamiliar disease. As a disease of voluntary muscles in older adults, slight weakening of a leg, arm, or hand; lessening coordination and tripping; or slight slurring of speech can easily be missed or attributed to advancing age. Once a diagnosis of ALS is arrived at, the concern becomes how to prepare the patient and caregivers and how to best manage the ordeal for all concerned. Each individual's disease progression is unique. Some appear gradually and progress slowly. Other individuals initiate more suddenly and then slow for a while at different stages. How and when do the most prevalent symptoms manifest?

EARLY STAGES

The symptoms of early stage ALS are relatively nonspecific, which often accounts for significant delay in diagnosis. For the two-thirds of the classical cases with the spinal form of ALS, they most often begin in the extremities, a foot or ankle that delays initiating movement or a hand that suddenly seems slow and weak or a localized loss of muscle mass. Usually only one extremity or body region is affected at first, followed by slow spreading of mild symptoms into contiguous muscle groups. In persons with onset of the bulbar form of ALS, which affects about one-third of all classical cases of ALS, the set of nerves that control the tongue, throat, face, and jaw are affected, causing the individual to experience slurring of speech and to have difficulties chewing and swallowing.

Muscles can be either weak and soft, or stiff, tight, and spastic. Uncontrolled cramping and twitching (fasciculations) can occur, and they can be painful. Individuals lose stamina and can fatigue easily while performing normal nonstrenuous everyday activities. They experience difficulties with balance and increased stumbling or tripping and falling while walking, due to unresponsive or weakly responsive muscles. This early phase of ALS can occur before a diagnosis of ALS is reached.

Middle Stages

In the middle stages of ALS, early symptoms become more widespread. Some weakened muscles become paralyzed, additional muscles are weakened, and fasciculations may remain while other muscles are unaffected. Muscle cramping and twitching affects arms, shoulders, and the tongue. Overall disability increases, and driving is discontinued. Balance is affected, falls are more common, and now the patient may require assistance to stand up. Muscles that can only twitch may permanently contract, and the prolonged shortening can produce mechanical strain on joints, causing pain and sometimes deformation of the joint.

Weakness develops in swallowing muscles (earlier in the bulbar form of ALS), causing choking exacerbated by excessive saliva accumulation and making it challenging to eat. The breathing muscles, especially those of the diaphragm, begin to weaken, making it difficult for the patient to breathe, particularly when lying down.

Difficulties in eating can lead to malnutrition, loss of body mass, and dehydration. Excessively low body mass, particularly rapid weight loss, in an ALS patient is correlated with more rapid functional decline and shorter survival. Weakened musculature causes poor posture, and the patient often experiences difficulty in holding their head up.

Behavioral changes may become more evident at this stage. It is not surprising that a patient realizing that they have an incurable fatal disease with a short survival time is likely to require emotional support and perhaps pharmacological assistance to avoid depression and withdrawal from those around them. In addition, a sizable proportion of patients have a component of frontal temporal dementia (ALS-FTD), which affects their behavior and requires additional treatment. Sleeping difficulties due to respiratory weakness, pain, anxiety, and depression are common.

Late Stages

At this point, most of the patient's voluntary muscles are paralyzed. The diaphragm and other respiratory muscles are severely weakened, making it very difficult for the patient to move air into and out of their lungs. This poor respiratory function lowers the oxygenation level of the blood, causing increased fatigue, dizziness, headaches, and decreased mental-processing ability. Eventually, respiratory dysfunction will require assistance, initially by noninvasive procedures and eventually, if agreed to by the patient, surgical (invasive) insertion of an airway tube. Speaking is impaired both by loss of control of the throat and jaw muscles and by the decreased mental capacity from low oxygen, and often by this stage, speech is completely lost. Communication shifts from verbal to writing or electronically enabled means.

While eye movements become abnormal, the extraocular eye muscles, which control eyeball movement, remain functional to a large extent for unknown reasons, as are sphincter muscles. Eating and drinking by mouth are severely impaired or impossible. Difficulties with coordinating chewing and swallowing make choking common and increase the possibility of the aspiration of food or drink into the lungs, leading to complications or fatal pneumonia.

Most Bothersome Symptoms Reported by Patients

Since ALS does not currently have a cure, treatment of the symptoms to improve patient quality of life is all that is available. There has been little critical assessment of patients regarding the symptoms that they experience, the treatments received for the symptoms, or the effectiveness of the treatments. This is not due to a lack of awareness of patient symptoms. A major reason is that there have been few high-quality studies (double-blind, placebo-controlled trials) of the effectiveness of symptom treatments in ALS patients. The processes causing the symptoms may be different in ALS from those in other diseases or conditions.

The lack of specific trials in ALS leads to the use of possibly ineffective therapies for treatment or inconsistent use of potentially effective ones. Many of the treatments are with off-label use of FDA-approved drugs, some of which insurance won't pay for. The lack of clinical trials goes back to the difficulties in financing trials in small numbers of patients with a rare disease, which has also impeded disease-modifying therapeutic development.

In order of those most frequently reported by patients in a large survey, the symptoms of ALS were fatigue, muscle stiffness, muscle cramps, shortness of breath, sleep difficulties, chronic pain, anxiety and depression, excessive saliva, constipation, pseudobulbar affect (swallowing/choking), loss of appetite, and weight loss. The survey did not evaluate the effectiveness of the treatments. The most bothersome of these reported symptoms were fatigue, muscle stiffness, and shortness of breath. The most troublesome symptom of all was fatigue. It also was the least frequently treated symptom. Other infrequently treated symptoms were weight loss, pseudobulbar affect, excessive salivation, muscle stiffness, and pain. The treatment of these symptoms will be covered in chapter 5.

CAUSES OF SYMPTOMS

Fatigue, the most common symptom reported by patients (44–83 percent), results from the cumulative effect of the long list of symptoms.

Physical fatigue rather than mental fatigue is most common in ALS, although depression can be a contributor. Dealing with muscle cramps and pain as well as the inevitable breathing difficulties also contribute.

Muscle stiffness, cramps, and spasticity are related symptoms, resulting from the uncoordinated activity of dying motor neurons innervating fewer and fewer muscle fibers and hyperactive reflex responses. This can be a significant source of pain in some patients and also limits mobility and function. Some patients report jaw quivering or clenching and cheek biting. This activity is due to spasticity triggered by pain, cold, or anxiety.

Shortness of breath, clinically referred to as *respiratory insufficiency*, is caused by the increasing weakness of muscles in the chest and the diaphragm. This weakness also impairs the cough response, which results in increased incidence of choking and aspiration pneumonia. Laryngospasm, the sensation that air cannot be breathed in or out for a period of seconds, is a frightening event for patients, because for a brief period of time, they cannot breathe or call for help. This can be caused by accumulation of saliva, acid reflux, or other liquid in the larynx (voice box) or triggered by other muscle-spasm inducers. While relatively uncommon in early stages of ALS, up to 19 percent of patients in later stages of the disease have experienced it.

Sleep disruption, like fatigue, is frequently caused by a variety of factors, especially respiratory muscle weakness but also pain, immobility, anxiety, and depression. Decreased sleep time leads to daytime fatigue and reduced quality of life, and it can have effects on prognosis.

Pain in ALS is not directly due to motor nerve dysfunction, because the sensory nerves responsible for sensing pain do not degenerate. Chronic pain is reported by 57–72 percent of ALS patients and is due to muscle immobility, weakness, cramping, and spasticity as well as joint immobility. Pain occurs in the neck, back, trunk, arms, or legs and can occur at any time during the progression of symptoms.

Anxiety and depression are experienced by many patients. Reporting of anxiety in ALS patients varies widely, ranging from 0–30 percent, and is more common early in disease progression, along with increased stress. The prevalence of depression in ALS patients is also widely variable depending on the assessment method.

Excessive saliva, or sialorrhea, is a condition in which saliva accumulates due to weakness of throat muscles involved in swallowing, giving rise to drooling. In ALS, sialorrhea is not an overproduction of saliva but an impairment of the normal process of saliva removal by swallowing. Up to 50 percent of ALS patients experience this condition. The pooling of fluid can lead to aspiration, infection, and pneumonia, which make it the second most common cause of death behind the failure of the respiratory muscles.

Edema, fluid accumulation in the hands and feet, occurs in ALS because of lack of mobility and muscle activity, which helps pump tissue fluids out of the limbs. Edema can result in burning sensations and leads to easily damaged skin.

Thickened bronchial secretions occur when weakness in the respiratory muscles that produce the coughing response impairs the expelling of mucus and other airway secretions from the lungs, causing choking and leading to pneumonia and other lung infections. Insufficient fluid intake due to difficulty in swallowing exacerbates the condition.

Constipation and urinary urgency due to gastrointestinal and urinary dysfunction have been reported in up to 29 percent of ALS patients. Reduced mobility of patients, decreased fluid and food intake, and side effects of medications contribute to these problems. Physiological changes in the spinal cord neurons responsible for controlling these functions weaken abdominal muscles for expelling stool and those required for urinary continence. ALS patients may need to urinate every one or two hours, and they are unable to move quickly to get to a bathroom. This further restricts their independence and opportunity for social interactions. Some patients will not leave their home because of their urinary urgency concerns.

Pseudobulbar affect, also known as *emotional incontinence,* is a behavioral condition experienced by 20–50 percent of ALS patients, especially those diagnosed with bulbar-onset muscular symptoms starting in the throat and jaw rather than an arm or leg. Patients may demonstrate sudden bouts of uncontrolled laughter or crying or other emotional outbursts that are unrelated to the situation and often do not reflect what they are feeling. It is distinct from a mood disorder, which has different cause. Involuntary crying is more common than laughing. These symptoms can cause significant disability, limit social interactions, and affect the patient's quality of life.

Loss of appetite increases as ALS progresses. Weakening jaw and throat muscles make it more difficult to chew and swallow, so less nourishment is consumed, which further weakens the musculature and creates a downward spiral. Reduced physical activity also requires less energy uptake, thus blunting appetite. Patient psychological depression also contributes to appetite loss.

Weight loss due to muscle wasting, as well as an inability to chew and swallow and a loss of appetite due to depression, is exacerbated by the overall hypermetabolic state of ALS patients. Additional energy is required to work weak muscles and to drive cramping, spasticity, fasciculations, and pseudobulbar behavioral symptoms. Loss of greater than 10 percent of body weight as well as rapid changes in body mass in the time from first symptom to diagnosis and within two years of being diagnosed with ALS are all associated with poorer prognosis. Conversely, mild obesity at diagnosis is associated with better prognosis.

IMPACT OF DELAY BEFORE DIAGNOSIS AFTER SYMPTOMS OCCUR

The lengthy delay in diagnosing ALS after report of first symptoms consistent with ALS occurs at a critical time for possible intervention in preventing or controlling spread of the pathology, leading to motor neuron and muscle fiber degeneration. Very early during symptom development, regeneration of nerve-muscle connections is attempted but then declines. Without its appropriate nerve and muscle target connections, the motor neuron dies. At that point, its associated muscle fibers no longer contract, and the muscle cells degenerate and die. The pathology continues to spread along regional neuronal connections.

While reversing this process is not currently possible, if appropriately targeted therapeutic interventions could be applied early enough, the extent of the damage might be limited and the progression of symptoms slowed or halted. The delay in diagnosing ALS dramatically narrows the window of opportunity for successful disease-modifying intervention. Identification of predictive biomarkers for presymptomatic phases of ALS could further improve the chances for such interventions.

The lack of presymptomatic biomarkers for ALS and the rapid progression of loss of function after the patient notices the first symptoms make it important that all patients and especially ones at risk for ALS, particularly genetic risk, seek medical advice when symptoms are first noticed. Delay between first symptoms and diagnosis of ALS complicates the management of functional changes. We will next consider the diagnostic process for differentiating ALS from other diseases with similar symptoms but different prognoses, treatments for symptoms of ALS, and management of the process.

5

Diagnosis, Treatment, and Management

The depiction of ALS as a relentlessly progressive, rapidly worsening of the paralysis of voluntary muscles until death is recognized by many neurologists. Converting this generalization to an orderly, consistent, systematic description for accurate diagnosis has been and continues to be a major challenge. The variability of presentation and prognosis, apparent multiple disease causes, and presence of clinical subtypes, as well as ALS-look-alike diseases, necessitate experienced, careful evaluation. Lack of predictive biomarkers severely hampers design and interpretation of clinical trials for effective treatments. It also impacts the management of the disease and increases the burden on the families and other caregivers.

THE STATE OF BIOMARKERS

A major void presently exists in the ability to detect the ALS disease process in patients before it is well advanced, producing the overt symptoms of muscle weakness and wasting. The 9–12-month delay between first symptoms and clinical diagnosis of ALS is a critical period in the progression of a disease with a survival time of only 2–4 years postdiagnosis. Lack of predictive and reliable biomarkers is a major obstacle to intervention clinical trials, because it lengthens trials, increasing expense and decreasing efficiency.

Primary outcome measures in ALS clinical trials are the survival or rate of decline, or both, on the ALS Functional Rating Scale–Revised (ALS-FRS-R). This requires lengthy trials before these robust measures become informative with respect to an intervention. One way around this obstacle is to use *biomarkers*, defined as surrogate objectively measured indicators specific or selective for and linked strongly to the primary clinical-trial outcome measures. No single test definitively diagnoses ALS. The earlier in the disease that biomarkers can be established, the more useful they will be, perhaps in early detection. These could include body fluid analyses, such as the blood tests to measure glucose levels as an indication of a diabetic condition or cholesterol levels as an indicator of risk for atherosclerosis. Cerebrospinal fluid biomarkers report on conditions in the brain, because of the connection with internal brain fluid. At present, the utility of biofluid (or wet) biomarkers in ALS is limited, consisting of different levels of a neurofilament protein that differentiate ALS patients from healthy normal subjects but not from other diseases.

Magnetic resonance imaging of upper motor neurons in the motor cortex of the brain is widely used to distinguish ALS from ALS mimics and from healthy control subjects. A specialized form of MRI called *diffusion tensor imaging* is able to distinguish groups of healthy controls from groups of ALS patients; it examines ALS-associated changes in brain-region pattern that follow disease progression. Unfortunately, the differences are not sufficiently large to be used to diagnose individual patients. The pattern of these changes is correlated with the pathological spread of disease and with ALS-FRS-R clinical-functional scores. Positron emission tomography (PET) imaging of metabolism in the motor cortex and certain other areas of differences in metabolic activity distinguishes symptomatic diagnosed ALS patients from healthy control subjects. How early in the disease process these methods are reliably informative of ALS remains to be established.

The main symptoms of ALS, those affecting muscle strength and respiratory function, are measurable and informative. However, they change relatively late in the disease course. Nerve conduction and muscle electrophysiology measurements are more sensitive than the clinical symptoms, but they are frequently confounded by the body's attempts to compensate for changes during progression.

CLASSIFICATION SYSTEMS FOR STAGING CLINICAL PROGRESSION OF ALS

ALS is the fastest-progressing neurodegenerative disorder and has the shortest survival time. An important component of managing a progressive disease is knowing after diagnosis where a patient is along the advancement time line. *Disease staging systems* have been in use for cancer for many years. They provide a simplified account of the degree of physical and functional characteristics of the disease affecting the individual, which aids caregivers in predicting patient needs. However, the variable presentation of ALS has made this somewhat difficult. Two complementary staging systems are currently in use: King's clinical staging, which follows the clinical or anatomical spread of the disease, and Milano-Torino functional staging, which measures the burden of dysfunction.

King's Clinical Staging

The King's system focuses on the number of body regions affected and recognizes five stages: presymptomatic, involvement of one, two, three clinical regions, and substantial respiratory or nutritional failure, prior to death. The King's system is more sensitive to changes early in the course of ALS.

Milano-Torino Functional Staging

The Milano-Torino system is based on the ALS Functional Rating Scale, a 48-point clinical measurement scale that assesses changes in four functional domains: bulbar (face, throat, and jaw), gross motor control, fine motor control, and respiratory measurements. The Milano-Torino system is more sensitive in later stages of the disease. The functional burden changes somewhat later than the clinical changes, due to muscle functional reserve in the region clinically impacted.

Neither of these systems currently takes into account the cognitive and behavioral changes that can present in a significant proportion of ALS patients. The Edinburgh Cognitive and Behavioral ALS Screen (ECAS) is used extensively, as it is highly sensitive in detecting deficits in diagnosed ALS cases. It is important to detect these changes in ALS patients, since cognitive and behavioral changes are associated with more rapid decline. Behavioral changes also place more of a burden on caregivers.

HOW ALS IS DIAGNOSED

ALS is diagnosed based on a combination of clinical observations, electrical measurements of motor neurons and muscle functional responses, and the exclusion of treatable disorders and ALS-mimic diseases.

Electrical measurements can detect physiological changes in both nerves and muscles. The Escorial clinical diagnostic criteria were developed originally in 1994 by the World Federation of Neurology Research Group on Motor Neuron Diseases. Subsequent revisions to these criteria, the Arlie House in 2000 and the Awaji-Shima in 2008, are agreed on by most experts. The Awaji-Shima criteria add results of tests for electrophysiologic abnormalities in nerve-muscle function on an equal footing with the clinical weakness observations. This increases the sensitivity for the detection of ALS.

The combined criteria are based on observed motor neuron-muscle weakness in four different body regions. Nerve-muscle electrical function testing, magnetic resonance imaging, and computerized axial tomography (CAT or CT) scans for structural changes, and positron emission tomography imaging for metabolic changes in nerves and muscles are used to rule out ALS mimics. The criteria were developed originally to facilitate research and the design of clinical trials. These Escorial criteria are not useful in all applications, and unfortunately the clinical terminology used to describe the clinical diagnosis can be confusing to patients. The diagnostic terms describe the conviction that the diagnosis of ALS is certain and that the patient does not have one of the other motor neuron diseases. The confusion comes from clinicians' use of the categories *possible, probable*, and *definitely* ALS. Patients tend to interpret them to refer to the certainty of the diagnosis of ALS rather than the severity of the clinical signs, which is the diagnostic meaning for clinicians.

Signs and Symptoms from Physical Examination

Although the disease process very likely began years earlier, it progressed silently for years, possibly decades in some individuals. It passed through a series of preclinical stages disabling normal biological functions driven by exposure to risk factors, genetic predisposition, and epigenetic changes. At some point, the cumulative effect of these changes leads to a short period in which electrodes inserted into the muscle can detect changes in the number of functional voluntary-muscle units and electrical-muscle activity. At this stage, these measurements can detect upper motor neuron dysfunction, while these measurements on lower motor neurons do not detect abnormalities, although this does not guarantee that these neurons are functioning normally. These muscle changes are still generally not noticeable to the patient.

The first symptoms patients notice can begin very subtly, with a single muscle, in many cases in a limb responding weakly or not at all. Unexplained stumbling or tripping while running, foot drop (weakness), or a walking motion with "slapping" of the foot on the floor due to poor muscular control are commonly reported by patients. With ALS, these changes are generally not accompanied by pain, since sensory nerves are not involved, although muscle spasms and hyperreactive reflexes can cause pain detected by sensory nerves. These muscle symptoms also could be caused by any one of a number of other neuromuscular diseases.

The main distinctive characteristic of ALS is its progressive nature and spreading to voluntary muscles in regions connected by motor neurons. Thus, following the progression during a series of examinations over a period of time is a key identifier in distinguishing ALS from a number of other neuromuscular diseases. Regular reevaluation is important if atypical factors are involved, such as pain or sensory changes. This verifying step is included because there are treatments for some of the other diseases, and prognoses for others are more benign than for ALS. Unfortunately, because of the generally rapid progression of ALS and loss of function, and only a 30-month survival after a lengthy ALS diagnosis process, there is less time to put in place interventions that might slow the functional progression or ease the burden of symptom management. This also complicates the design of clinical trials, particularly ones aimed at processes occurring earlier in the disease progression.

Diagnostic Testing—Excluding Other Diseases

Diagnostic testing is carried out on several levels. Since there is currently no accepted laboratory testing that will diagnose ALS by itself, laboratory testing beyond the clinical observations for ALS is primarily exclusionary. Metabolic, nutritional or toxic disorders, structural lesions or damage, infection, a number of hereditary diseases, tumors, vascular lesions, nerve-muscle connective disorders, and muscle diseases can all cause symptoms that also occur in ALS. Testing is performed early in the evaluation of an individual for ALS, because many of these tests are useful in detecting other muscle diseases before the typical ALS patterns and spreading of loss of muscle function can be clearly identified.

Electrical Activity of Muscle Fibers—Electromyography

Lower motor neuron loss, which accounts for two-thirds of classical ALS cases, can be readily measured by electrodiagnostic techniques. The simplest measurement of muscle function is muscle strength using an instrument called a *dynamometer*. However, for ALS patients, although dynamometer testing is easy to perform and reliable, because it is measuring a late process of the disease, it is not very useful as a predictor. *Electromyography* is a different technique that measures the electrical properties of the muscle. Surface electrodes or thin-needle electrodes inserted into the muscle can measure the normal resting electrical activity of the muscle, the activity from voluntary movement of the muscle, as well as the bursts of activity arising from spontaneous muscle twitching (fasciculations) that are a feature in ALS. Surface-electrode measurements are sensitive only to muscles close to the surface.

Electromyography with needle electrodes can be used to assess the number of active motor units in a muscle. A *motor unit* is the number of muscle fibers in a muscle innervated by a single motor neuron. Both the number of motor units and size of the motor unit (number of fibers responding) can be estimated. These measurement parameters progressively decrease with the disease.

Nerve Conduction Studies

A different type of measurement is called *nerve conduction*, in which a nerve is electrically stimulated with an electrode and the response of the muscle that it innervates (is connected with) is measured. For ALS, motor neuron–muscle connections are monitored by measuring the time for the stimulating signal to reach the muscle as well as the size of the muscle response. The size of the response decreases with time and disease progression. The process of motor neuron reinnervation of muscle fibers in an attempt to maintain connectivity interferes with the ability of this method to monitor motor neuron loss. Weakness, as measured clinically, is only apparent after a significant number of motor neurons are lost.

Loss of upper motor neurons, those involved with the muscles of the face and throat, are much more difficult to measure by electrodiagnostic methods, especially if their effects are interfered with by dysfunction of the lower motor neurons. Bulbar ALS, affecting upper motor neurons accounts, for one-third of the classical ALS cases. A nonimaging method called *transcranial magnetic stimulation* excites neurons in the brain motor cortex, in which upper motor neurons reside, and the response is measured in a hand (innervated by upper motor neurons). MRI structural imaging and more sophisticated MRI and metabolic PET methods may prove useful in distinguishing patients with ALS from normal and from ALS mimics. These diagnostic methods are currently being optimized for use in ALS.

Electrodiagnostic measurements can reveal nerve-muscle changes that occur before muscle function deterioration is noticed by the patient, but they can appear coincident in time. Changes in nerve-muscle communication are not restricted to ALS. A major reason the measurements are performed as part of the diagnostic workup is to distinguish or rule out other myopathies (muscle diseases). These have different prognoses and treatments to be considered later in this chapter.

Magnetic Resonance Imaging

Modern imaging of the living nervous system provides a major advance in detecting structural, physiological, and functional changes in remarkable detail. While X-ray imaging (CAT scans) provides detailed structural information of the skeletal system and other denser structures in the body, magnetic resonance imaging offers structural and functional information about soft tissue, such as the brain and nerves. It can detect degeneration of nerve tracts, such as those connecting the motor cortex and bulbar region in the progression of ALS and other diseases.

It also can monitor structural and functional changes in the connectivity between different regions in the brain extending beyond the motor system that are responsible for the clinical manifestations of ALS, including cognitive impairment. The locations of these changes distinguish potentially ALS-relevant processes from those causing other diseases. Magnetic resonance imaging is useful for diagnosing ALS and distinguishing it from other diseases, but since it is not sensitive to the earliest changes in ALS, it is not useful for early stage diagnosis.

Tests for Other Disorders That Share Some ALS Symptoms

General blood work checks glucose and electrolyte levels and measures liver function or damage. Different tests are required for ALS. Creatine kinase enzyme activity in the blood is a general feature of brain and muscle damage. Vitamin B12 determinations will reveal deficient vitamin levels, which can cause metabolic defects leading to anemia and neurological symptoms. Motor neurons are particularly sensitive to low vitamin B_{12} levels. Low copper levels can also lead to blood disorders and neurological symptoms. Deficiency in copper is frequently found in combination with vitamin B_{12} deficiency, as both can result from nutritional deficiency. Unfortunately, these tests are not specific for ALS.

Neuropsychological Testing

If ALS is a motor neuron disease, why is there concern about something that seems so distant from voluntary muscle control as cognition and behavior? It has been only in the past 25 years that studies have confirmed that more than the motor system was involved in ALS. In the past 10 years, researchers have been able to put some patient numbers to this association. Nearly 50 percent of patients diagnosed with ALS have some form of cognitive impairment, and 10–15 percent eventually meet the baseline criteria for frontotemporal dementia.

As a result, a whole new diagnostic category was defined, amyotrophic lateral sclerosis-frontotemporal dementia. A specific type of FTD, the behavioral variant (bvFTD), is associated with ALS. Bulbar onset ALS has been more directly connected with cognitive impairment. This is not very surprising, considering that the motor cortex region of the brain and the upper motor neurons involved in bulbar onset ALS are situated physically close to the frontal and temporal brain regions affected in FTD and may share some connectivity. In FTD and ALS-FTD, similar protein deposits composed of the misfolded TDP43 protein are the classical pathological features observed on autopsy.

The cognitive deficits in ALS affect different functions than the more well-known and dramatic memory loss seen in Alzheimer's disease. In ALS, the cognitive features that are affected most strongly are the type called *executive functions*. They help with decision-making, planning, strategizing, motivation, and controlling responses (inhibitory control). These deficits can alter a patient's day-to-day abilities. Verbal fluency tests have to be adapted to the difficulties bulbar onset patients experience with jaw and facial muscle movement. Language deficits, independent of executive function, are also common in ALS and are similar to those seen in FTD, including naming, word relationships, and meaning.

Overlapping with FTD, ALS-FTD patients have impaired social understanding, poor judgment of person-to-person interactions, emotional lability (rapid extreme changes in mood), and an inability to judge other people's state of mind in order to predict others' responses. The proportion of ALS patients who show apathy can reach 80 percent. Agitation, aggression, and a lack of empathy have all been observed with both FTD and ALS. Hallucinations and delusions are infrequent in FTD, but they are emerging as presenting symptoms of ALS-FTD.

Behavioral Diagnostic Testing

Verbal fluency evaluation, which tests the number of words in a subject category a person can verbally list, is sensitive to executive function deficits that can identify patients needing more comprehensive testing. The cognitive screens originally established for FTD can be employed as long as the physical disabilities of the ALS patients are taken into account. Screens specifically designed for ALS, such as the ALS-Cognitive Behavioral Screen (ALS-CBS) and the Edinburgh Cognitive and Behavioral ALS Screen, are used most often. The ALS-CBS focuses on the executive function and is less sensitive to nonexecutive functions such as learning and long-term memory, while ECAS addresses several cognitive domains besides executive function.

Functional MRI and PET neuroimaging have been used to detect abnormalities in brain regions associated with executive dysfunction and emotional processing, but these remain research studies at present and do not provide a dramatic improvement for diagnosis over the performance of neuropsychological testing protocols.

Ability to Make Medical and End-of-Life Decisions

The early detection of cognitive impairment in a significant proportion of ALS cases, those eventually diagnosed with ALS-FTD, has dramatic consequences for management of the patient's care during both the functional decline and terminal phases of the disease. A prominent feature of the type of cognitive decline is that while FTD does not affect memory like Alzheimer's disease, it strongly influences decision-making, planning, and strategizing, precisely those abilities that require the best judgment when making medical and end-of-life decisions. The diagnosis of ALS-FTD primes family, caretakers, and the treatment team to take into account the eventuality that the patient will not be able to effectively take part in some decisions. Early diagnosis will allow time for those involved to come to grips with the situation and to plan for the future.

Genetic Counseling

Because ALS is a rare disease and strongly influenced by many genes with small individual effects as well as by variably influential environmental risk factors, genetic studies focus on the single gene-driven familial forms of ALS, which account for around 10 percent of all cases. In a patient already experiencing symptoms consistent with ALS, knowing about a pathological mutation in a gene or genes can provide perspective on prognosis and assist in the planning of patient care and symptom management. Because of uncertainties in how the genetic component may be expressed, presymptomatic genetic testing of family members in families with a history of ALS is controversial, and routine testing is recommended to be undertaken only in specialist centers.

However, in order to conduct research to reconstruct the pathways by which ALS is initiated and progresses, it is important that at-risk individuals be identified and their disease process studied. The most accurate way of identifying at-risk individuals is using those genetic mutations that can be traced in families and most consistently drive fALS with similar features. By following these individuals presymptomatically, researchers can begin to determine a series of steps or stages in which changes occur and lead eventually to symptoms. By targeting events in the different stages, treatments may be found that will slow or interrupt the previously relentless progression of the disease into a symptomatic phase.

In order to perform genetic testing on individuals, counseling is required to ensure that patient participation is voluntary, that confidentiality is protected, and that informed consent is obtained. Genetic counseling consists of a series of sessions with a support person. In a research center, counseling is provided before any decisions are made to proceed with the testing; such counseling describes what consent is and is also provided in a series of pretesting and posttesting sessions. In the predecision consenting counseling session, the individual's reasons for wanting to undergo genetic testing are explored. This includes perceived benefits of the testing and personal lifecycle timing, such as starting a relationship or a family. It also provides the opportunity to detect the presence of coercion by a family member or by researchers.

Evaluation of the individual's psychosocial readiness to undergo testing is performed. This includes assessing risk factors like psychiatric conditions, current substance abuse, presence of risk factors for suicide, and absence of a social support system. After each session, written summaries of verbal communications are provided to the individual, and adequate time is allowed for assimilation of the material, including additional counseling sessions, if requested. In the pretest counseling session, issues about psychological effects, the presence of an appropriate support system, and concerns about insurance coverage are explored. At any time, the patient may stop the process and not proceed to testing. Testing results are to be provided within a reasonable time frame.

Posttest counseling takes place in the presence of a friend or family member. Immediately before disclosure, it is confirmed that the individual feels ready to receive the testing results, and then the findings are communicated. The potential clinical and psychological effects for the individual of knowing these results are discussed, along with the implications for the family. The limitations of current genetic testing as they apply to ALS and the uncertainties—what we know and do not know about the disease—are explained. Finally, resources for the individual and family are identified.

Familial ALS

Cases occurring in families where there is a history of ALS are considered familial. Until recently, because of the overall rarity of ALS, the criteria were if at least two biologically related members of a family had ALS, the cases were considered genetically driven and designated fALS. The disease was considered sporadic (sALS) if only one person in the family had ever had ALS. For various reasons, including ancestral origin, there are many reasons why a family history may not be clear cut.

Even for family members who have the same mutation in the same protein, because of different experiences between individuals and other genetic interactions, there is no guarantee that they will become symptomatic or follow the same disease course. Unlike some other neurodegenerative diseases, such as Huntington's disease in which the type of mutation is highly predictive of age of onset and prognosis, the impact of any given mutant gene in fALS is somewhat uncertain. Although there are clear potential patient benefits of genetic testing to identify individuals carrying a mutation considered a genetic cause of ALS, because of the uncertainty and personal reasons, individuals have the right to choose not to know their genetic status.

Sporadic ALS

In cases where sporadic ALS is suspected because there is no family history, genetic testing is less predictive than in fALS with a family history. All of the genetic mutants found in fALS have also been found in (apparently) sporadic ALS. Because of the current primitive understanding of diseases where mutations in a few genes have a major effect on the disease process but do not always cause the same effects, learning that a given mutation is present in an individual is not all that helpful in predicting progression or responses to treatments.

ASKING FOR A SECOND NEUROLOGICAL OPINION

The uncertainty of diagnosis is disconcerting to many patients. A second neurologist's independent opinion may be requested, in addition to ruling out alternative diagnoses or accessing alternative treatments.

MOTOR NEURON DISEASES THAT RESEMBLE ALS BUT HAVE DIFFERENT OUTCOMES

The onset of ALS-like symptoms can be very subtle. This may mean that a patient is in the early stages of developing classical ALS. Since ALS is a uniformly fatal disease, the physician will want to be as sure as possible before delivering a diagnosis and will follow the progression of symptoms. Another reason for delaying a diagnosis of ALS for further testing is a number of other motor neuron diseases symptomatically resemble ALS. Sometimes called *ALS mimics*, these other diseases are individually rarer than ALS, but they have different, less draconian outcomes, which makes it important that they be diagnosed properly. Whether it is ALS or one of the mimics, the best chance for impacting the rate of progression is in the earliest symptomatic stages. The opportunity is lost or the effect of an intervention is decreased as time passes.

Progressive Muscular Atrophy (PMA)

PMA, also known as Duchenne-Aran muscular dystrophy, is the most common of the ALS mimics, representing 4–11 percent of all motor neuron disease cases. It is a sporadic (nongenetic) disease sometimes confused in the literature with spinal muscular atrophy, which is a recessive genetic disorder (see below). PMA has a prevalence of 1.7–4.2 per 100,000 living individuals, depending on the ethnicity of the population studied. In distinction to ALS, PMA lacks the hypersensitive reflexes, spasticity, and emotional lability frequently seen in ALS.

There is some controversy over whether PMA is a different disease affecting motor neurons or simply a variant of ALS. Symptoms initially appear in muscles controlled by lower motor neurons (brainstem, spinal cord) in the legs. At later times, upper motor neurons (brain motor cortex) may become involved, producing symptoms in arms, face, and jaw. Age at diagnosis is 30–60 years old, the same as ALS. Duration can be many years, and importantly the 5-year survival rate is 56 percent, compared to 14 percent for ALS.

Primary Lateral Sclerosis (PLS)

PLS is a slowly progressing, sporadic upper motor neuron disorder with symptoms of weakness and spasticity in all four limbs; it accounts for about 4 percent of all motor neuron diseases. The mean age of onset is 59 years, and the 10-year survival rate is 71.1 percent.

Spinal Muscular Atrophy (SMA)

SMA is an inherited motor neuron disorder resulting from a mutation in the survival-of-motor-neuron (SMN) gene on chromosome 5, which results in the death of anterior horn cells located in the spinal cord, affecting lower motor neurons. The incidence of the disease is 8 per 100,000 live births, which may be an underestimate due to fetal death, and a prevalence of 1–2 per 100,000 living people. There are five forms of this motor neuron disease. Symptoms can appear any time from birth to adult. The infantile form, called *Werdnig-Hoffmann disease,* comprises 45 percent of cases and is fatal by 1–2 years old.

Adult forms of the disease (age of onset 20–50 years) progress very slowly over decades. Adult onset SMA is much less incapacitating than the juvenile forms. Adults experience weakness in the legs, torso, shoulders, and upper back. It progresses very slowly, with normal or close to normal life expectancy, and only a small proportion end up requiring a wheelchair. The 10-year survival with the adult form of SMA is 100 percent.

Spinobulbar Muscular Atrophy (Kennedy Disease)

Spinobulbar muscular atrophy, or Kennedy (Kennedy's) disease, is an inherited progressive muscle disorder affecting the androgen (male hormone) receptor gene on the X chromosome. Like SMA, it affects the anterior horn cells of the spinal cord and lower motor neurons, but unlike SMA, it affects only males. Since the gene is on the X-chromosome, the disease affects males mostly in their thirties and forties, with a prevalence of 1 in 30,000 male births and an incidence of 0.2–0.7 in 100,000 males. Very few women are affected, probably due to their low levels of testosterone, the hormone whose action is mediated through the androgen receptor (mutated in Kennedy disease).

Mainly the lower motor neurons are affected as in SMA, although in some patients, upper motor neurons are affected. Symptoms occur at 20–50 years old and are concentrated at 30–40 years, beginning with facial muscle twitches, followed by weakness and hand tremor at onset. Patients continue to develop general muscle weakness in their arms and legs, and they experience difficulty swallowing and talking. Life expectancy ranges from slightly diminished by 10–15 years to normal, although about 10 percent of patients die in their sixties or seventies, due to aspiration pneumonia resulting from difficulties swallowing. A blood chemistry characteristic of Kennedy disease is a greatly elevated creatine kinase level, an enzyme released by damaged brain and muscle.

OTHER DISEASES WITH SIMILAR SYMPTOMS TO BE RULED OUT

Several diseases or syndromes also have muscle weakness as a major symptom but are not ALS. Many of the tests are not diagnostic for ALS but are to identify other diseases in order to design an effective management plan and to detect other diseases and their variants that may be treatable.

Although not an exhaustive list, several of the more commonly encountered conditions are briefly described here. A number of them include autoimmunity as their underlying mechanism, which is not the case with ALS.

Myasthenia Gravis

Antibodies produced by the individual patient target the acetylcholine receptor on the muscle. They prevent the signal released by the lower motor neuron, acetylcholine, from being received by the muscle. The reason for the production of these antibodies is not understood. As the levels of the antibodies in the body fluctuate, so does the weakness of facial muscles controlling chewing, talking, facial expressions, and slurred speech, among others. Overall weakness and ease of tiring of legs, arms, hands, and fingers is also present. Diagnosis is based on the inability of the patient to perform repetitive muscle contractions or simply hold their arms outstretched for a minute. Even though the motor neurons are spared, electromyography measurements show decreasing muscle response upon repetitive electrical stimulation.

Myasthenia gravis is slightly more common than ALS, and it is more common in women, with diagnosis between the ages of 20–40 years, while men are most commonly diagnosed at over 50 years of age. Life expectancy is normal, although the patient's quality of life can be compromised.

Lambert Eaton Myotonia

Lambert Eaton myotonia is another autoimmune condition in which antibodies attack a membrane protein that triggers motor neurons to release the acetylcholine neurotransmitter. This myotonia is observed in cases of certain cancers, small cell carcinomas, as a side effect of the immune system trying to battle the nonmuscle cancer cells, which have a similar membrane protein. Frequently the neurological symptoms appear first as weakness in the arms and legs, and the cancer is detected later. Unlike myasthenia gravis, repetitive stimulation of the nerve or use of the muscles actually gradually *strengthens* the muscle response, because with multiple stimulations, there are more chances for the acetylcholine to be released, and the acetylcholine receptor on the muscle is intact. The disease is treated by targeting the tumor with chemotherapy and radiation to reduce the immune response.

Lambert Eaton myotonia is much rarer than ALS, with an incidence of three or four cases per million. While it can occur at any age, it is most prevalent in smokers over 40 years of age, which is consistent with the cancer connection.

Guillain-Barré Syndrome

Guillain-Barré syndrome is a syndrome rather than a single disease, because it presents in a variety of ways. It develops in response to a gut viral infection or, rarely, after vaccination. Progressive weakness appears over a period of 2–3 weeks, and then in most patients, it resolves spontaneously. As a response to the infection, the patient's immune system produces antibodies that attack the insulating myelin sheath around the motor neurons disrupting the signal conduction to the muscle, although the reason for this is not understood. Although 70 percent of patients recover in 6–36 months, 30 percent have residual muscle weakness.

TREATMENTS: THE DEVELOPMENT OF THERAPEUTICS

The type of study design for sensitively testing an intervention's effectiveness is called a *randomized controlled trial*. In the simplest version, patients are assigned at random to groups, *control* (treated with an inactive substance, a placebo) or *treatment* (treated with the substance being tested for therapeutic activity). The responses of the two populations are compared for effects on symptoms or on biomarkers, such as a blood test. In certain trials, the placebo and treatment groups are then switched so that the placebo group gets treatment and the treatment group gets placebo, and then the responses are compared. Some version of these designs is required for maximum sensitivity, although the specific parameters very much depend on the particular disease.

Current Understanding of the Disease Process and Future Clinical Trials

Several possibilities have been suggested to explain the lack of progress in finding effective therapeutics for ALS. While Charcot's development of an archetype descriptor for ALS consolidated clinical observations and improved diagnosis, the heterogeneity of the disease evident in the numerous variants lumped together as ALS may be part of the difficulty. ALS has been characterized as a syndrome, which is actually a family of clinically similar disease states with potentially different biological mechanisms. The clinical spectrum of ALS is complex. Symptoms initially develop in different areas (legs, arms, face) with different severity, spread differently, and progress at variable rates to final stages.

A major difficulty is that currently diagnosis of ALS is determined from clinical symptoms. By the time clinical symptoms manifest, it is already late in the pathogenic process, and many motor neurons have degenerated. Knowledge about the mechanism(s) leading to motor neuron degeneration is fragmentary and uncertain. Biomarkers specific for ALS, particularly disease variants that are detectable before symptoms appear, are virtually nonexistent. Add to this the genetic complexity of ALS, even in the familial heritable forms, which produce dominant effects. Multiple genes leading to clinical ALS produce different outcomes for different mutations within the same protein. In the sporadic forms of ALS, there are also contributions from groups of genes associated with ALS that on their own do not cause ALS.

There is no lack of human clinical trials ongoing, initiated, or in some stage of progress on ALS treatments. A database provided by the U.S. National Library of Medicine of private and publicly funded studies in 202 countries and all 50 states can be accessed at www.clinicaltrials.gov. Out of over 1,000 studies listed, there are hundreds of ALS trials in various stages, and new ones are constantly being added. The testing process is slow and extremely expensive. Most are small trials to test safety, looking for promising effects on aspects of ALS on symptoms or less often due to expense progression of the human disease. They are not the definitive large trials needed to support approval by the Federal Food and Drug Administration that signify real progress towards a possible therapeutic.

FDA-Approved Drugs

The Federal Food and Drug Administration is the U.S. federal government agency responsible for certifying premarket review of the safety and therapeutic efficacy of all new drugs. Just two drugs are currently approved for treating ALS. There continue to be ongoing trials of potential drugs for ALS.

Riluzole (Rilutek)

Originally called Rilutek, riluzole was approved by the FDA in 1995 and went generic in 2013. The drug targeted the degeneration of motor neurons. A common cause of motor neuronal death is hyperactivity with the neurons firing abnormally. Riluzole has a number of effects on aspects of glutamate neurotransmission activity that result in the reduction of over-excitation of neurons that use glutamate, including motor neurons. Besides in ALS, it is used in instances of spinal cord injury to reduce glutamatergic nerve-cell death and in a number of other nervous system conditions. Clinical trials with riluzole showed that the agent was most protective in extending life span by 3–5 months if started early in the symptomatic clinical course. Its major effects on life span are noticeable later in the disease course, and time to hospitalization is lengthened.

Riluzole is expensive, although the generic can be considerably cheaper. Both Medicare and the Veterans Administration cover it, and the National Organization for Rare Diseases can help cover costs for the indigent. Riluzole is taken by mouth (originally available in tablet form) and is most effective when combined with comprehensive symptomatic treatments. In 2018, the FDA approved an oral suspension form of riluzole developed by ITF Pharma, Tiglutik, for use in the United States. The suspension is designed to be more easily used than tablets by ALS patients who have difficulty swallowing. Riluzole treatment does not work for everyone. The magnitude of efficacy is disputed, and some countries have not approved the use of riluzole.

Edaravone (Radicava)

Edaravone (Radicava) was approved by the FDA on May 5, 2017. It is targeted at free radicals, highly reactive chemicals produced in neurons and other cell types during metabolism that become toxic and cause degeneration when there is an imbalance in protective mechanisms. Following safety testing first in animals and then in humans, the drug's effectiveness was evaluated in a randomized, double-blind, parallel-group study in a limited set of cases of ALS or probable ALS that also met certain other criteria. Starting studies with as homogenous a patient group as possible increases the ability to observe drug effects.

After 6 months, treatment scores on the ALS Functional Rating Scale–Revised showed a 33 percent reduced rate of decline. The study did not test whether patient survival was extended or whether ALS patients not meeting the strict criteria for inclusion would benefit from the drug. It is likely that additional studies with modified criteria will determine if patient survival is lengthened and whether a larger proportion of the spectrum of ALS patients can be helped by the drug. An oral dosage form is not available. Edaravone is administered intravenously in 28-day cycles (14 days on the drug; 14 days off). It is a very expensive drug for the uninsured.

Potential Therapies in the Pipeline

In an age where antibiotics can clear a microbial infection completely and insulin treatments can normalize diabetic conditions, the very limited treatment effects of ALS drugs are highly disappointing. A similar lack of effective therapeutics for other neurodegenerative diseases like Alzheimer's and Parkinson's diseases, despite multiple clinical trials, also bedevils progress on those diseases.

Many potential therapeutics for ALS have been tested and failed to demonstrate significant magnitude of effects on disease symptoms, disease progression, or survival time. Like many clinical trials, early testing included a number of initially promising candidates. When evaluated in randomized control trials, the best controlled study design to detect moderate-sized therapeutic effects, those initial results could not be replicated. Although animal model studies, performed on familial ALS gene-modified mice, had been supportive, there was no demonstrable effect in humans, most of whom were believed to have sporadic ALS rather than the much rarer familial forms of the disease.

The compounds tested were chosen because they acted on pathways shown to be affected in both sporadic and familial forms of ALS. Mechanisms included regulators of overactive glutamate neurotransmitter activity of motor neurons, trophic factors that support motor neuron health, supporters of neuronal energy production by the cellular mitochondria powerhouses, antioxidants, and stimulators of the degradation of protein aggregates that accumulate in motor neurons.

Complementary and Alternative Therapies

Because ALS has such a devastating prognosis and there are no cures or evidence-based, clinically meaningful disease-modifying treatments that significantly slow the progression, there are a host of strategies used by physicians and caregivers to ease the burden for ALS patients. Some behavioral approaches, such as meditation training and active music therapy, have been tested in randomized controlled clinical trials. Symptom management has improved over the years, but desperate patients and caregivers often reach out on the internet for possible solutions even if there is no medical proof that they work. In fact, such treatments may cause problems of their own, interfering with the limited effects of available therapeutic approaches by being substituted for those approaches. A number of alternative and complementary approaches most commonly applied are mentioned here.

Diets and Nutritional Supplements

The strongest and most effective strategy for lengthening survival is maintaining weight and caloric intake. Unlike the healthy individual in today's society where a reduction in caloric intake promotes health, in ALS the opposite is true; extreme weight loss and often emaciation are common and can accelerate progression. Some of the effect is energy imbalance, and this is exacerbated in forms of ALS where chewing and swallowing are affected, causing insufficient calories and inadequate nutrition to be consumed. There is controversy over what kind of hypercaloric diet is best, high carbohydrate or high fat, although both diet forms appear to be safe and reasonably well tolerated.

A variety of nutritional supplements have been suggested based on their effects on biological processes altered in ALS. Vitamins (vitamin A, vitamin B_{12}, vitamin C, vitamin D, vitamin E, thiamine, riboflavin) either show no effect or have not been rigorously tested in humans in clinical trials. Regulators or intermediates in cellular energy production like creatine, L-carnitine, and Co-Q10 address the deficit of energy production in ALS. Of these, only L-carnitine (as acetyl-L-carnitine) has been demonstrated in a randomized double-blind placebo-controlled pilot study to extend ALS patient survival and reduce some symptoms. Natural products like catechins, found in fruits, vegetables, and green tea, and resveratrol, found in in red wine, are protective of cellular processes affected by free radical damage of the type seen in ALS. However, no effects on progression or symptoms of ALS have been demonstrable in clinical trials.

Cannabis

Cannabis, a mixture of over 400 chemical compounds found in extracts of several *Cannabis* plant species, has been reported to be useful in controlling symptoms, particularly pain, excess salivation, depression, loss of appetite, and muscle spasticity. Some active components are a group of 60 or so compounds called *cannabinoids*, which target the natural regulators of a pathway in humans and other animals that impact biological processes driving the symptoms. Other cannabis components are not psychoactive and can regulate some of those same pathways.

Chelation

Exposure to heavy metals (lead, arsenic, mercury) through drinking water or as an occupational environmental hazard of mining has been considered a risk factor for ALS, because of a correlation of an increase in ALS prevalence with working in mining or living in areas with mining-contaminated water sources. However, there is no consistent evidence showing that exposure to heavy metals causes ALS. Chelating agents bind heavy metals in the body and cause them to be excreted in the urine. There is no evidence that treating with chelating agents has any effect on the clinical course of ALS, nor have heavy metals been detected in the urine of ALS patients treated with chelating agents.

Acupuncture

The traditional Asian technique of inserting thin needles at certain locations (acupoints) has been used for millennia to achieve therapeutic effects. Although the clinical mechanism of acupuncture is not well understood, there is some evidence that two symptoms of ALS, pain and spasticity, can be alleviated by acupuncture, although the effects can be modest. Beyond this, clinically significant effects are palliative, and no effects on disease progression or survival have been demonstrated in clinical trials for ALS.

Energy Healing

The effects of this form of alternative medicine, which also includes spiritual and faith healing, have been studied by randomized, placebo-controlled trials in multiple diseases. All of these studies have failed to show any significant effect on disease symptoms or progression. Although no trials on energy healing in ALS have been published, ALS forums contain many reports of the significant financial cost but lack of benefit of energy healing practices on ALS.

Treatment of Symptoms

Although therapeutics capable of major effects on the progression of the processes driving the disease are currently not available, palliative measures can provide some measure of control of symptom intensity and have an impact on improving the quality of life of ALS patients.

Symptom treatments have been borrowed from those used for other disease states, due to the lack of solid controlled clinical trials for effectiveness in patients with ALS. These include pharmacological interventions when applicable, as well as physical and psychological assistance addressing the features of the underlying disability. Because the circumstances surrounding the symptoms are not necessarily the same as in other diseases, strategies that work for other diseases may not be effective in ALS. For example, pain in one disease is not necessarily caused in the same way, nor does it routinely respond to the same pharmacological or nonpharmacological treatment in another disease state. The therapies that are applied are in line with good clinical practice in general, but they don't always accomplish the desired result in ALS patients.

Nonpharmacological Treatments

Because treatment for ALS is largely palliative, intervention begins with nonpharmacological modalities in an attempt to mitigate symptoms. Physical therapy, such as stretching and range of motion exercises, especially those involving the shoulders, helps to keep those joints flexible and to prevent the pain of contractures and the ensuing joint deformation. Some small research studies indicate that moderate exercise employing

ALS-suitable levels of low-impact activities, such as light resistance training, cycling (stationary bike), and exercises in a pool balanced with breaks throughout the day, can be beneficial. The feedback of activity on weakening muscles can slow the denervation process and allow patients to more effectively use assistive devices like walkers and wheelchairs. Discretion is advised, and avoiding overexertion is important in preventing acute pain, fatigue, and soreness.

Pharmacological Treatments

If symptoms don't improve with nonpharmacological treatments, then pharmacologic measures are introduced. A combination of pharmacologic and nonpharmacologic treatments is often required to reduce the severity of symptoms. Pharmacologic agents, drugs, are classified by their biological target, which is likely to be causing or amplifying different symptoms. *Anticholinergics*, which block the action of the neurotransmitter acetylcholine, are often used to treat sialorrhea (excess saliva) and to control urinary urgency and frequency. Brand-name anticholinergic drugs like Ditropan, Oxytrol, Detrol, Vesicare, and Enablex have been used in the United States for the treatment of ALS symptoms.

Antidepressants and a*nxiolytics*, as their names suggest, work to control depression and reduce anxiety that contributes to almost all of the symptoms of ALS. These include pseudobulbar affect, weight loss, sleep difficulty, sialorrhea, muscle cramps and spasticity, jaw quivering/cheek biting, and fatigue. Commonly used brand-name antidepressants, which include several different subtypes, are Zoloft, Prozac, Paxil, Effexor, Cymbalta, Wellbutrin, and Remeron. Brand-name anxiolytics include Xanax, Ativan, Valium, and Klonopin. Antidepressants and anxiolytics can help control instances of behavioral changes and to strengthen patient's coping skills. Caregivers can also suffer from depression and anxiety with all of the pressure of caring for the patient, and that can also affect their overall health.

Pain medications range from opioids like morphine and Fentanyl for refractory pain to nonopioids. Nonopioids include acetaminophen, and nonsteroidal anti-inflammatory drugs, such as ibuprofen (Motrin, Advil), Celebrex, or Cambia, are used for milder pain.

The types of treatments and interventions used to treat common symptoms are described below in the order of the frequency of symptoms reported by ALS patients.

Fatigue, from the constant effort of breathing and dealing with the muscle cramping and chronic pain, is combated by an overall attempt to conserve the patient's energy level and by addressing the stressors individually. A practical approach is pursued, employing strategies to alleviate the symptoms, and may include nonaddictive stimulants. Fatigue can also be due to depressive processes and be responsive to antidepressants and anxiolytics.

Muscle stiffness, from lack of use and patient immobility, can be relieved by physical therapy, including stretching and range-of-motion exercises.

Muscle cramps and spasticity are treated by careful physical stretching and range-of-motion exercises as well as by massage and hydrotherapies, such as water jets, hot tubs, and whirlpool baths. Pharmacological treatments include benzodiazepines and muscle relaxants. The latter agents should be monitored to prevent excessive muscle weakness. Jaw quivering or clenching and cheek biting can be treated with benzodiazepines.

Shortness of breath, or respiratory insufficiency from the progressive weakening of muscles responsible for breathing in the chest and the diaphragm, is the main life-limiting symptom of ALS. Pulmonary function should be assessed every 3–6 months in order to monitor the need for noninvasive ventilation. When the total amount of exhaled air (forced vital capacity) declines to 50 percent of normal for the patient or the maximal inhaled pressure of air (maximal inspiratory pressure) is less than a minimum depending on the patient, noninvasive respiratory assistance is recommended to extend survival and to slow the decrease in the volume of air the diaphragm can pull into the lungs. This volume is critical to providing enough oxygen and removing carbon dioxide from the bloodstream in the lungs.

The decision with its pros and cons to undertake noninvasive ventilation (NIV) and/or its more invasive intervention, a tracheostomy with surgical implantation of a breathing tube, should be discussed with a pulmonologist or respiratory therapist expert with managing neuromuscular disease patients. In this discussion, the opinions and wishes of the patient and family should be paramount. At this time, it is also prudent to discuss subjects like drawing up a living will and a durable power of attorney for health care and to update these documents if necessary.

Sleep difficulties are caused by disruptions of sleep time due to symptoms leading to fatigue such as depression, cramps, pain, and breathing difficulties. As respiratory function declines, episodes of inadequate oxygen and buildup of carbon dioxide wake patients more often, and sleep time suffers, increasing fatigue. NIV can significantly improve sleep time by normalizing ventilation. A motorized hospital bed can facilitate patient repositioning and enhance mobility, as can adjustable mattresses. Encouraging behaviors that promote good sleeping habits, such as scheduling activities around a fixed sleep schedule, can minimize disruption of the patient's sleep cycle. Antidepressants can reduce the contribution of depression and anxiety to sleep disturbance, as can anxiolytics if used selectively, although intervening in the underlying causes for anxiety is to be preferred.

Chronic pain has no specific treatments. Physical therapy interventions that move and gently stretch weak or immobile muscles in order to prevent contracture formation, move joints, and reduce muscle spasms have different effects on individual patients. Providing an alternating pressure mattress to reduce immobility or even simply changing cushions on chairs can have a dramatic effect. The use of orthotic devices to mechanically support weak limbs and joints can reduce pain. Nonopioid and opioid analgesics, nonsteroidal anti-inflammatory drugs (NSAIDs), and muscle relaxants are used, taking care to avoid excessive muscle weakness.

Anxiety and depression symptoms can be alleviated by psychotherapy and counseling. They can also address the deeper psychological effect of being diagnosed with a fatal rapidly progressing disease that suddenly takes away the ability to move, communicate with others, and breathe. A number of different approaches may be helpful for ALS patients, such as relaxation strategies employing methods like meditation and biofeedback. Cognitive behavioral therapy teaches patients skills to adjust their thinking in order to avoid sliding into an unproductive mental state and to realign their emotional state. Anxiolytic and antidepressant therapeutics have been described to treat the contribution of these mental states to the multicomponent symptoms in ALS.

Excessive saliva, or sialorrhea, is the accumulation and pooling of normal saliva production due to the loss of the ability to properly swallow, as the throat muscles weaken. A major concern for many ALS patients, it can become an agent of significant mortality if it is aspirated into the lungs because of poor throat muscle strength and control, where it can form a focus of infection and cause pneumonia. As a first line of defense, saliva production can be reduced by anticholinergics, although this approach may not be sufficient to block this symptom. An alternative is using a suction device to periodically extract the accumulated saliva from the throat. Finally there is salivary gland ablation, in which the salivary glands are inactivated by radiation or surgery. More recently, injection of the glands with botulinum toxin type B, an agent used cosmetically to reduce facial wrinkles, blocks the acetylcholine-stimulated release of saliva from the glands.

Thickened bronchial secretions, primarily mucus coating the airways and other airway secretions from the lungs, accumulates due to the weakened coughing strength of the respiratory musculature. This material is mechanically removed by suction, and when that is insufficient pressure-driven assistive lung inflation and emptying devices (sufflators) are used. Proper patient fluid hydration, room or NIV device humidity control, and pharmacological mucus liquefiers (mucolytics) to reduce the viscosity of mucus and other secretions increase the effectiveness of these devices. This system also allows for the clearance of secretions in individuals who also have respiratory tract infections, which can be a problem in ALS cases with aspiration pneumonia.

Constipation and urinary urgency occur when weakened abdominal muscles prevent effective voiding of stool. Increased dietary fluid and fiber intake supplemented by fiber laxatives and a recommended amount of water can relieve the constipation, which is then followed by control of fiber and fluid intake and laxative control. Nutrition adjustment is through diet or tube feeding. Treatments of last resort for constipation are enemas and manual impaction removal. Urinary urgency can be controlled or adapted to by scheduled voiding, avoidance of caffeine and alcohol, use of a urinal, and catheterization. Anticholinergics can be used after urinary tract infections or an enlarged prostate have been ruled out. Medication efficacy depends on the individual patient.

Edema, fluid accumulation in the hands and feet due to immobility, is treated mainly by elevation of the limbs above the level of the heart and an adjustable hospital bed. Passive range of motion, moving of the legs, and stretching exercises all can help redistribute the excess fluid. Compression stockings are difficult to put on and take off. Since fluid load is not the difficulty in ALS, diuretics are avoided, as they exacerbate cramping.

Pseudobulbar affect is a behavioral condition that is most frequent in ALS patients with bulbar onset of muscular symptoms characterized by episodes of involuntary uncontrolled laughing or crying not reflecting the feelings of the patient. This emotional lability is not considered a mood disorder, but the symptoms respond to certain neurotransmitter uptake inhibitors (serotonin reuptake, tricyclic antidepressants, serotonin-norepinephrine reuptake) that are effective in treating mood dysfunction. A combination of dextromethorphan/quinidine (Nuedexta) has been approved by the FDA as a treatment.

Weight loss in ALS patients is a profound characteristic of the disease and is not restricted to loss of muscle mass. There is abundant evidence that ALS is accompanied by a change of metabolic state from normal to a hypermetabolism, which is associated with greater functional decline and shorter survival. Treatments center around making up for the additional metabolic turnover, since it isn't clear where the energy that should be invested in maintaining body mass is going, and requires making up for reduced patient appetite related to depression and to the gradual decrease in appetite during disease progression.

Appetite stimulants can help some with this, but they are not a long-term solution. After a nutritionist evaluation, introduction of snacks, more frequent meals, and high-calorie supplements can help stabilize body mass for a while. Difficulties experienced with chewing and swallowing can be addressed by eating changes, such as smaller bites, slowing eating, and avoiding talking. As the symptoms progress, changing the consistency of the food by blending solid food and adding thickener to liquids can help. There is evidence for the effectiveness of enteral nutrition through a gastrostomy feeding tube in stabilizing body mass.

The above treatments are suggested as good clinical practice and are commonly used. Palliative, they are intended to make the patient as comfortable as possible. They don't generally significantly change the course of the functional decline, and the effectiveness varies with the patient. Physicians as well as patients are not satisfied with the effectiveness of current palliative treatments.

Enhanced Nutrition

Most of the palliative treatments described affect the ALS patient's quality of life but exert little influence on survival time. One possible exception to this is nutrition. Rapid weight loss, predictor of a shorter survival time, occurs in patients due to increased nutritional demands from an increased metabolic rate, as a result of losses in muscle mass and nutritional losses of fat and nonfat body mass. The reasons for this are not well understood. Slowing of weight loss by nutritional supplements combines both high-caloric content and nutritional adjustments to supply ample vitamins and minerals. These adjustments can alter the rate of decline of functionality in individual patients, but they cannot in the end prevent the final stages of the disease and death.

Assistive Technologies

In the very earliest stages of ALS, the individual may ask for assistance while engaging in certain tasks that have become challenging or frightening. It is helpful to provide emotional support and to adapt the environment for as much independence as possible while protecting the safety of the individual and others around them. Simple assistive devices, such as a cane or a leg brace, may be useful by helping preserving mobility.

Occupational therapists can help make activities of daily living easier for the patient through maximizing mobility and comfort by adapting activities and by patient and family education. This can be seemingly as simple as recommending certain clothing and modifications like particular shoes and laces, button and zipper aids, special writing tools, and keyboards. Along with physical therapists, occupational therapists can prescribe assistive equipment like wheelchairs and walkers, communication devices, leg braces, and hand and wrist splints. which become more helpful with increasing disability. Shower chairs improve hygiene, lift chairs and rising toilet seats help patients get up, and transfer boards and mechanical lifts help with transfer from one place to another. Noninvasive breathing assistance can improve sleep quality.

A variety of technologies is available to assist the ALS patient with their activities of daily living and with maintaining critical physiologic functions, in particular breathing. Some of the equipment may be obtained on loan from *equipment closets* maintained by various organizations that reuse devices provided by families of former patients or purchased with donated funds. Stocks of assistive equipment are essential, because a patient's needs can change suddenly. Obtaining insurance approval/reimbursement and delivery of new equipment, particularly if some modification is required, can take a significant amount of time and is expensive. Loaned equipment can help bridge the gap.

Mobility

Ways to support the needs of patients to supplement their mobility and, eventually, communication needs are increasingly provided by technologies. The most basic mobility assistance comes from braces, walkers, lifts, and other types of physical support, transitioning to wheelchairs, either manual or eventually motorized, when walking is no longer possible or dangerous. Customized wheelchairs can be tailored to help individuals get around, to stand, and to sleep, but they take time, often months, to produce and can cost $25, 000–$30,000.

Communication

To take advantage of assistive technologies, the patient needs to be able to communicate with the devices and with other people. Communication devices, essential later in the disease process, include device adaptations that allow any patient-controlled movable body part to operate communication devices and other equipment. They are the last link for the patient to communicate with caregivers and family. At first, the voice strength weakens, so amplification is useful to allow the patient to be heard. After the voice fails, writing can be either by hand or with the assistance of eWriters, an electronic writing instrument. Text-to-speech applications using smartphones or other electronic devices can also be employed for audible communication. Eye-gaze-controlled technology is increasingly available for a number of devices both in communication or for patient-initiated activities in later stages, as eye movement is relatively unaffected in many ALS patients.

Biomedical engineering adapted to specific physical conditions is increasingly helpful to people with different types of disability. Numerous devices being created and tested could ease the effect of ALS symptoms on quality of life. Speech-generating devices can be produced for an individual's state of disability, and some can be adapted to adjust to the disease progression. Stephen Hawking, the physicist, used a computer system to synthesize a voice to talk for him for years, which he operated with a single muscle on his face that he could still control. Finding one that works for an individual patient may not be easy. In many areas, off-the-shelf devices for an individual are not available, and they can be expensive. Custom-built devices can also take a long time to build and can be difficult to adapt as the individual patient declines.

Respiration

Sustaining respiratory function in the face of the loss of the diaphragm's voluntary muscular control is used to extend the life of the ALS patient, most of whom die from respiratory failure or complications resulting from swallowing issues leading to aspiration pneumonia. There are both noninvasive and surgically invasive procedures available to provide adequate respiratory function. The decision to use these methods and the timing of their use to prolong life is something for the patient to decide, communicate to caregivers, and document while still able to do so. *Diaphragmatic pacing* involving stimulation of the diaphragm muscle in ALS patients reduces sleep apnea, in which breathing stops for a period of time during sleep; however, use of this pacing technology is associated with reduced patient survival time.

Noninvasive ventilation, the most common form of respiratory assistance for ALS, involves a mask that the patient wears and does not include an invasive artificial airway, such as an endotracheal tube or tracheostomy. Pressure-support ventilation assists the weakened diaphragm and other respiratory muscles to take in a breath (inspire) with positive air pressure when triggered by the patient's attempt to breathe. Breathing out is triggered by the slowing of the rate of air intake. The patient can adjust the trigger points for these processes to be most comfortable.

Patients with ALS with bulbar dysfunction often have swallowing difficulties and an inability to cough productively to remove mucus and other obstructions that, if not managed, can lead to choking and aspiration pneumonia. Once an ALS patient loses the ability to clear airway secretions, noninvasive ventilation is no longer a viable treatment option, and the decision for either surgical intervention or palliative treatment has to be made.

Either *noninvasive or invasive respiratory assistance* is used to provide respiratory sufficiency for as long as the patient agrees. For those patients who choose to undergo surgery when the noninvasive ventilation is inadequate or their respiratory muscles have failed, surgical insertion of an endotracheal tube by tracheostomy is an alternative. This is often the final stage of respiratory assistance beyond which palliative treatment is currently the only option. Discussion about the use of respiratory assistance among the patient, caregivers, and medical staff needs to take place before the patient loses the ability to communicate verbally and while the patient is mentally able to make decisions (a major concern in cases of ALS-FTD). The patient also should have the option to change their mind about these near end-of-life decisions.

MANAGEMENT OF ALS

Once symptoms start, functional decline begins to progress in a relatively linear fashion as voluntary muscles gradually lose their motor-neuronal input. Along the way, symptoms can appear abruptly as the body struggles to maintain control of muscle activity and increasing imbalance in excitatory and inhibitory inputs causes spasticity and cramping with associated muscular pain. Each patient's course of disease is different in detail because of the many factors that come into play during progression.

The different types of symptom presentation and the rapid pace of changes compared to many other diseases can be overwhelming to caregivers, family, and the patient. It is therefore important that planning for management of patient care be considered even before diagnostic testing is complete, ready to put in place as soon as possible after the diagnosis of ALS to deal with the impact of the information. A well-thought-out *management plan* provides the best foundation for being able to keep up with the multitude of changes coming up and increasing the ability to head off and to deal with expected and unexpected difficulties. The goal of case management is twofold: to improve the patient's quality of life as much and for as long as possible and to decrease the stress on caregivers.

Most people with ALS will need treatment from a broad spectrum of both medical and mental health care providers. The most effective integration of this *multidisciplinary treatment team* is through specialist clinics dealing with ALS. Team members include a neurologist, rehabilitation physician, physical therapist, occupational therapist, respiratory therapist, dietician, neuropsychologist, speech therapist, nurse, and social worker. Not all are required all the time, but they need to be kept updated so that they are ready to rapidly step in at any time. This multidisciplinary team is as much for the caregivers as for the patient.

In the absence of this team, coordinating the scheduling of multiple different specialist providers, getting them to communicate effectively, and transporting the patient to appointments is an overwhelming task. Having to keep up with the details will have a negative effect on the patient's mental and physical state and will soon burn out the most well-meaning caregivers. Additional team members like home health care providers, a medical equipment specialist, and an assistive technology specialist may be called upon, depending on the patient's health needs. The goal of all this is to keep the patient healthy and safe, as well to maintain the patient's independence for as long as possible and to help caregivers cope with the situation.

Issues

Major issues to be addressed beyond palliative symptomatic care include personal decisions by the patient on how much or whether certain treatments they are willing to undergo, where they feel most comfortable living, how much assistive technology to use and, which kind, if any, when noninvasive and mechanical ventilation support is acceptable, and finally, what sort of end-of-life preparations they want. ALS strongly impacts family members and others with an emotional attachment to the patient. They face a grueling physical and mental ordeal assisting with the care of their loved one, including how they will deal with the patient's expressed choices for treatment or nontreatment, which may not coincide with their personal outlook.

Treatment Options

The treatment options for ALS are mostly palliative, treating the symptoms to minimize patient suffering as they appear. Some prophylactic efforts, like proper nutrition and trying to limit weight loss, are the most effective at extending survival. Breathing support as required in the later stages also prolongs survival. The FDA-approved therapeutic armamentarium for ALS is limited to riluzole (Rilutek) and, more recently, edaravone (Radicava), which may add a few months to survival. Other therapeutic possibilities include enrolling in a clinical trial of a potential therapeutic. Alternative therapeutic avenues of different types abound. They should be approached with care and with the guidance of a physician familiar with ALS, as these treatments have not been demonstrated to be effective in rigorous clinical trials. This may seem to be a debatable argument for a disease with no cure. The main concern here is to avoid treatments that could aggravate symptoms or bring on more difficulties for the patient.

This chapter has described the diagnosis of ALS, treatment options, both the limited FDA-approved therapeutics targeted to slow disease progression and palliative therapies intended to alleviate symptoms, and the management of a treatment plan. We will next consider survival-time prognosis for patients with different forms or subtypes of ALS and will address the reality of living with a person with ALS, including general management of their care.

6

Long-Term Prognosis and Potential Complications

ALS is presently not a curable disease. It is also a baffling disorder in many ways because of its heterogeneous presentation in individuals. Its symptoms can resemble multiple other diseases or conditions involving neuromuscular systems, such as those described in chapter 5. Many of these can be treated with some success or have less dire consequences. Hence, the great investment of time and effort that physicians spend to accurately diagnose ALS.

SURVIVAL TIME

Within ALS, some themes for prognosis have been recognized, and they are generally associated with the rate of progression of functional decline and survival time. Different clinical presentations correlate overall with different survival times. However, it needs to be emphasized that individual patients vary greatly in their presentation and rate of progression. The themes are derived from patterns observed in the statistics from group analysis of large numbers of patients.

Numerous studies have followed clinical signs like respiratory function or biomarkers, such as albumin, creatinine, and neurofilament protein levels in body fluids. The overall average survival time for ALS is 3 years postdiagnosis. However, 20 percent of patients live for 5 years, 10 percent live for 10 years, and 5 percent can live for 20 years or more. What these studies cannot do is provide precise information about the outlook for an individual patient. Predictions generated from published studies can be extremely unreliable in predicting the outcome for individual patients.

Death comes to most ALS patients quietly in their sleep. Progressive weakening of the diaphragm muscles decreases the volume of air moved into and out of the lungs. The resulting increasing carbon-dioxide levels and lower oxygen content in the blood at some point leads to a loss of consciousness and death.

As ALS progresses, weakening and loss of muscular control of the jaws, tongue, throat, and diaphragm combined with excess salivation causes difficulties in coordinating chewing, swallowing, and breathing. These symptoms are prominent early in cases of bulbar onset ALS, which initially affects these muscles. Along with the accumulation of phlegm and mucus in the throat, the loss of control leads to choking and aspirating food, saliva, and drink into the lungs, which then are susceptible to bacterial or viral infection leading to pneumonia, another leading cause of death for ALS patients.

Factors Predicting Longer Survival

Limb dysfunction, rather than speech or swallowing (bulbar) dysfunction, is often associated with longer survival times. So is symptom onset at an early age rather than middle age. The physicist Stephen Hawking was 21 when he was diagnosed with ALS, but he lived to age 76. His continued research in cosmology and theoretical physics amply demonstrated that he did not suffer from cognitive impairment, such as in ALS-FTD. Presentation with mainly flaccid weakness of arms or legs on both sides of the body, known as flail arm or flail leg, or upper motor neuron variants of ALS have prognoses with 5-year survival rates over 50 percent. The best indicator of slowest progression is a long interval between symptom onset and clinical diagnosis, likely because of the slower overall progression of the disease process.

Factors Predicting Shorter Survival

Forms of ALS with cognitive impairment, but not necessarily full-blown ALS-FTD, with symptoms concentrated in executive function affecting cognition, behavior, or emotion and suggesting involvement of the frontal lobes of the brain have poorer prognosis. The reasons for this are not well understood at this time.

Other indicators of poor prognosis are rapid diagnosis soon after first symptoms presentation or rapid weight loss before diagnosis. Respiratory involvement, although not necessarily respiratory onset before other symptoms, also is linked with poor prognosis. Survival times associated with these other indicators can be as short as 12 months.

Genetic Factors in Prognosis

Familial forms or specific nonfamilial genetic risk factors (mutations) associated with ALS can also affect survival times. Multiple different mutants of SOD1 are capable of causing ALS, most of which reduce survival time. Different mutants of the SOD1 gene that change single amino acids in the protein sequence of SOD1 affect the disease prognosis. The Asp91Ala variation of the SOD1 gene is associated with very slow progression, while the Ala5Val variation at a different position in the same SOD1 protein is associated with very rapid progression. Again, the reasons for these differences are not understood. Other genetic variations in other, nonfamilial ALS genes, such as UNC13A and CAMTA1, also affect survival duration.

Rates of Progression for an Individual: Implications for Care

Both the sequence of symptoms emerging as ALS develops and the rate at which functionality decreases often differ between individuals. In addition, for any particular individual, progression can slow down, speed up, or even seem to stop for a period of time. Very rarely the overall symptoms can improve somewhat, but they inevitably return relatively quickly. These changes make it difficult physically and mentally for the patient, as well as for the caregivers and the health care professionals to deal with. This volatility makes it imperative for there to be a coordinated and adaptable plan in place to manage the care.

PLANNING FOR AND LIVING WITH ALS

The key to minimizing the trauma to the ALS patient and caregivers is in learning what to expect and the organizing and accessing of resources for both patient care and support of caregivers in ways that are applicable to the individual family situation. This includes working at some level with multidisciplinary healthcare professionals to deal with the specific issues of in-home care, as well as managing practical issues such as the financial burden through insurance and governmental and nongovernmental agencies, and the legal issues of advanced directives concerning the decision-making competence of the patient and end-of-life decisions.

Staging of Care

The amount and type of care needed for a person diagnosed with ALS depends on their stage in the progression of the disease and the specific effects on that individual. The proportion of care provided by the family caregivers and medical and other professionals also depends heavily on the individual and the disease stage.

In early stages of the disease, symptoms may be weak or spastic muscle cramping and loss of muscle mass which causes fatigue. Behavioral changes include poor balance, tripping while walking, slurred words, and dropping things due to weakened grip. These symptoms may be restricted to a single body region or may occur mildly in several different regions. This stage can already be present before diagnosis. When asked, caregivers provide help with some tasks, including offering a cane or a leg brace, and emotional support. They should look to adapt the physical environment to maximize patient safety and independence and to share the news of the diagnosis of ALS with children, relatives, and friends. It is also time to review and update legal, medical, financial, and other plans and to explore government (veterans) and insurance benefits.

In middle stages, the symptoms spread to connected areas. Some muscles are paralyzed, others weakened, while others remain unaffected. Joints may become rigid, painful, and sometimes even deformed. Driving is discontinued, which restricts social interactions and is a harbinger of the personal mobility changes to come. Weakness in swallowing muscles can cause choking, trouble eating, talking, and problems handling saliva. Respiratory problems may begin, especially when lying down. In ALS-FTD cases, uncontrolled laughing or crying inappropriate to the situation can occur.

At this stage, it is more common for patients to need active assistance in preserving a measure of functionality. Range-of-motion exercises help keep joints from seizing up. Braces and splints stretch extremities and maintain positioning. Adaptive equipment (wheelchairs, communication devices, shower chairs) becomes important. Lift chairs and toilet seats, as well as lift boards and mechanical lifts, provide safer transfers for both patient and caregivers. Declining physical function eventually requires feeding tubes to prevent choking and help maintain weight, and noninvasive ventilation helps with weak breathing.

Caregivers, who are often family members, should ask for help from others in providing the physical assistance needed with eating, drinking, toileting, bathing, and other affected functions. As those in closest contact with the patient, caregivers evaluate standing, walking, and swallowing abilities and, with input from medical personnel, adjust for safety. By involving the patient in matters of day-to-day living, decision-making, and planning, caregivers can be on the watch for signs of patient depression and can alert the physician. As a result of this responsibility, caregivers need to be aware of the toll it takes on them, keeping a close watch on their own health, particularly for depression and anxiety, and to work with the physician to identify coping strategies.

In late stages, most patients' voluntary muscles are paralyzed. Respiratory function is extremely compromised, and mobility is very limited. The weak respiratory function can lead to pneumonia. Eating and drinking by mouth and speech may no longer be possible. Assistive devices directed by any moving body part may be required (power wheelchairs, hospital beds, mechanical lifts, computers, communication devices, environmental controls). Either noninvasive respiratory measures or invasive tracheostomy may be required, as may a feeding tube. Urinary catheters may make toileting easier, although they may not be required. At this stage additional caregiving help may be needed to assist with 24-hour care. Establishing a routine and finding ways to keep the patient as socially and mentally active as possible help to maintain patient quality of life.

Organizing Care

If this seems an overwhelming experience, it is. While some people deal with the multitude of issues that ALS presents with a minimum of health care assistance, the best and least traumatic experience for the caregivers and the patient requires a coordinated team approach, including contributions from other personnel as well as physicians.

In-Home Care

Many ALS patients are cared for at home, especially those who are not able to leave home. This is frequently with the aid of home visits by members of a multidisciplinary team, who provide assistance and guidance on home safety, supportive counseling, education, training in the use of assistive devices, evaluation and fitting of loaner assistive equipment, and end-of-life planning.

Health Care System

The multidisciplinary team approach to ALS is offered by many hospitals, Veterans Administration medical centers, and health care facilities around the United States. Depending on location, some clinics operate full-time, while other specialty clinics are available through scheduled visits. Specialty certified centers and care clinics work with the ALS Association (www.alsa.org) and the Muscular Dystrophy Association (www.mda .org) to treat ALS. Patients and caregivers can use the websites of these organizations to locate specialty clinics in their geographical area.

Additional information is available through the ALS Therapy Development Institute (www.als.net), the National Institute of Neurological Disorders and Stroke of the National Institutes of Health (www.ninds.nih.gov /Disorders/Patient-Caregiver-Education/Fact-Sheets/Amyotrophic-Lateral -Sclerosis-ALS-Fact-Sheet), and Project ALS (www.projectals.org). A number of these websites have programs where they lend used and donated medical equipment to patients for little or no charge.

Support for Caregivers and Family

In the multidisciplinary team approach, both patients and caregivers appreciate a proactive involvement of a case manager in anticipating future care needs and discussion of procedures, as well as the emotional support in dealing with the many needs of the patient and the stress of caring for a loved one, often a spouse or other family member. Caregivers often place the well-being of the patient above their own. To a certain extent, this is understandable, but it is not a sustainable situation, as a stressed caregiver is not as capable of providing care at the level the patient needs. Both parties suffer the consequences. It is therefore to the advantage of both the patient and the caregiver that counseling and respite be provided for the caregiver. Indeed, if not explicitly provided, caregivers should seek that necessary help and not be concerned that they will be thought weak.

Supportive Care

Within the context of the multidisciplinary team approach, supportive care addresses a multitude of needs at the levels of the individual patient and caregivers. The number of clinical and nonclinical specialists involved can be bewildering to both the patient and the family caregivers. A nurse provides the connection between the patient and the treatment team and also provides assistance where needed in implementing aspects of multiple parts of care. The following describes the components of an individualized treatment plan with a brief description of the specialists involved and what they offer as part of the team.

Psychological Support and Behavioral Management

A *clinical neuropsychologist* monitors the patient's cognitive, emotional, and behavioral function, caring for mental health in general as well as assessing for possible dementia. This is particularly important if the patient has been diagnosed with ALS-FTD, which involves brain areas controlling cognitive and behavioral functions in addition to the motor cortex region, which controls voluntary muscle movements. Neuropsychologists also will provide supportive therapy for caregivers as well as suggest treatment for patient emotional issues associated with ALS, such as uncontrolled laughing or crying.

Medication

A *neurologist*, a physician whose specialty training focuses on the brain and the nervous system, directs and manages the overall medical treatment plan. This includes developing the plan and amending it as the patient's situation evolves. Treatment for the ALS disease process, such as riluzole, will be prescribed, as well as other pharmacological and nonpharmacological treatments to manage the ALS symptoms, such as excessive salivation, cramps, stiffness, and emotional lability.

Physical and Occupational Therapy

A *physical therapist* and an *occupational therapist* endeavor to optimize daily living by implementing strategies that will maintain the patient's mobility and independence to the greatest extent possible. They educate the patient and caregivers about strategies for the use of personalized exercises and adaptive devices, such as manual and power wheelchairs, braces, and shower chairs. A *rehabilitation physician* prescribes the specialized equipment as needed for walking, balance, and moving around at home and out in the community. The occupational therapist offers strategies for improving the daily living activities of eating, toileting, bathing, and dressing.

Nutritional Support

Weight management and proper nutrition are important parts of care planning for ALS. The rate of weight loss of the patient is highly correlated with the rate of progression of the disease and functional decline. A team comprised of a *gastroenterologist, dietician*, and *nutritionist* develop a plan to monitor and maintain proper daily caloric, vitamin, essential-nutrient, fat, and protein intake in order to maintain as constant a weight as possible. They advise on food type and consistency, when swallowing and choking become major issues, and for the need for placement of a feeding tube. The insertion of a feeding tube requires a surgical procedure performed by a gastroenterologist.

Swallowing Support

A *speech therapist* assesses and follows the changes in the patient's ability to chew, swallow, drink, and speak. When swallowing becomes difficult, the speech therapist implements a variety of types of assistive approaches to help the patient eat and drink. The speech therapist will discuss the placement of a feeding tube, when the chance of choking while swallowing becomes dangerous because it could lead to aspiration pneumonia, a common cause of death for ALS patients. By working with the dietician, the speech therapist can adjust the consistency of the food to make chewing and swallowing easier.

A *speech language pathologist* will monitor the patient's speaking ability and, in conjunction with the speech therapist, will offer strategies to for improving communication and the use of devices to assist or augment communication. Having a person who keeps track of the rapid advances in communication-device technology and methods, their applications, and efficacy can help maintain that tenuous connection with the patient when the options for communication would otherwise dwindle.

Breathing Support

A *pulmonologist* will work with a *respiratory therapist* to educate the patient and caregivers about how ALS affects breathing. They assess changes, such as shortness of breath during the regular movements required for eating, bathing, talking, or lying down. Their goal is to maintain breathing independence for as long as possible.

Education, Counseling, Community Resources, and Programs for Patient and Caregivers

Social workers provide information on how to manage nonmedical aspects of caring for an ALS patient, including financial, insurance, and legal assistance. Importantly, they can advise on the availability of a variety of local community resources and programs for the patient and for caregivers, as well as employment, transportation, and home-care issues.

Lifestyle Changes

When amyotrophic lateral sclerosis strikes an individual, the effect on all members of the family unit is profound and far-reaching. Few diseases are as relentlessly and rapidly progressive or more uniformly fatal as ALS. It cannot help but traumatize family and friends to watch a loved one slip away, losing many of their personal characteristics and eventually become totally dependent on others for the tiniest details of living.

Patient

The patient increasingly loses the ability to move and engage in physical activities. Everything comes to a halt; careers are interrupted, and future life plans dashed. Eventually, normal bodily functions like chewing, swallowing, and breathing are compromised. All the while, the patient's cognitive abilities are relatively unaffected (except for some of those with ALS-FTD), so they know what is happening to them and feel powerless. They are entirely dependent on others to do the simplest things for them.

This helplessness is bound to have negative effects on the patient's outlook on life, their emotional stability, and the way they feel about themselves. This often also becomes an issue for the caregivers, who are trying their best to cope with the situation. The patient realizes that they are a burden on their family. In this situation, the best a patient can do is to communicate their wishes about how far caregivers and the multidisciplinary health care team should go with palliative care, especially in the later stages of ALS involving respiratory and life support.

Caregivers

Most caregivers of an ALS patient are members of the family, frequently their spouse, which makes the stress and strain of having to deal with ALS more acute. Family caregivers face a doubly difficult situation. A loved one is stricken with an incurable disease that progressively worsens, and the caregivers are in the front lines every day with the patient as they deteriorate. They have to do things they never thought they would ever have to do and need to plan ahead for the inevitable. At the same time, they try to put the best face on all of this with the patient.

Interaction with the multidisciplinary health care team is essential for training in caregiving, since this is not often a role that family caregivers have had to take on at this level. Asking for help, not just with procedures but with coping mechanisms for the stress and strain of caring for a family member with an incurable fatal disease, is essential.

Family and Friends

In addition to the prospect of losing a family member to ALS, the time and intensity of commitment to caring for a patient with ALS is stressful for families. It is most extreme for the immediate family members who are involved in patient care or interact frequently with the patient, but even more distant family relationships can be affected. Since ALS can be familial, there may be some concern about the possibility of others in the family developing ALS.

Friends want to help but are unsure about their place in the situation or ways they could help. Many families turn inward to deal with catastrophes of this magnitude, but they could benefit from the help of friends, who could help with transportation of the patient to medical appointments or simply relieve caregivers by being with the patient. Religious civic organizations could also provide assistance of this type to relieve the burden on the primary caregivers.

Financial Burden

The cost of treating ALS derives from medical services as well as loss of income from both the patient as well as the caregiver(s), because the task of caregiving, transporting to clinical appointments, and arranging for day and night supervision expands to fill their whole lives. Both commercial private insurance and Medicare, since many ALS patients are old enough to be on Medicare, shoulder a substantial portion of the financial burden of caring for an ALS patient. However, there are significant out-of-pocket expenses that can be a burden for many families additionally stretched by the loss of family income from the patient and from caregivers, who are often a spouse.

Cost of Treatment and Management

In the United States, a study published in 2015 using commercial insurance and Medicare databases for medical costs and a survey of families for nonmedical costs (adapting housing and paid caregiving) arrived at a figure of $63,693 per year per patient (medical costs alone were $31,121 per year). This yielded calculated U.S. population-wide costs for 2010 of $1.023 billion, based on population prevalence of ALS. These are costs averaged over the course of the disease. Costs rise significantly with increasing patient disability. Caring for individual patients can cost significantly more, depending on circumstances and insurance coverages. Costs also differ between different countries for a variety of reasons, and the United States is on the high end of costs.

Insurance Coverage

In the United States, insurance coverage is often the responsibility of the individual, and the extent of that coverage depends on the individual case, except where the patient is covered by Medicare. Countries like South Korea have a national health insurance system for rare and intractable diseases, which includes ALS. The coverage rate is 90 percent, but there are still considerable out-of-pocket costs for treating ALS in such systems.

Legal Assistance

The social worker provides information about a wide variety of non-medical issues for the ALS patient and caregivers. While not directly advising on these issues, they provide access to the relevant local information sources on specific topics. They advise on finding help on financial issues, disability insurance, and different services. They are also aware of the need for planning in the organization of legal issues concerning the patient, who at some point will be unable to execute decisions on matters like living wills, durable powers of attorney, hospice, medical insurance, and end-of-life matters.

Primary among these, a *living will* is a form of advanced directive prepared while the patient is legally competent to make decisions that provides guidance on medical and health care decisions, including withdrawal of life support and the level of palliative care; it is used when the patient becomes no longer competent to make those decisions on their own. This is particularly important for ALS patients, who will likely be unable to talk or physically communicate their desires to their caregivers or medical personnel. Also, a significant proportion of cases of ALS have some form of ALS-FTD, in which the cognitive processes are affected, rendering patients mentally incompetent to make decisions as well as physically unable. In different jurisdictions, the legal standing of a patient's wishes as expressed in advanced directives also varies, so it is important that there be appropriate local legal arrangements.

END-OF-LIFE MANAGEMENT

At the point when respiratory function in an ALS patient becomes severely compromised, noninvasive ventilation has been shown to extend survival. However, when a patient can no longer tolerate NIV or it is no longer effective, the remaining options are few. Discontinuing NIV and simply maintaining supportive symptomatic care with specialist services is one option with relatively short-term survival prospects. Alternatively, invasive mechanical ventilation with tracheostomy surgery and insertion of a gastrostomy tube is chosen by some patients. While survival time is not necessarily increased by this intervention, patient quality of life can be improved, the risk of rapid loss of weight and of dehydration avoided, and patient anxiety can potentially be reduced. Meanwhile, however, the disease process continues to advance with increasing loss of independence and communication ability.

Although most ALS patients express a preference to die at home, the advanced stages of care are extremely complicated, difficult to deal with, and expensive to support at home, leading to hospice, nursing-home, or other institutional care. The use of the invasive ventilation procedure varies among countries and is influenced by the differences in culture, the type of health care options and systems available, and applicable law. As a result, individual patients do not all have the same access to life-prolonging but high-expense care options.

Although many ALS patients fear choking to death, it is actually rare and mostly associated with individuals with severe bulbar symptoms. The vast majority die peacefully in their sleep.

This chapter describes the prognostic factors associated with longer or shorter patient survival time with ALS. It delves into management of ALS with the assistance of a multidisciplinary team of health care professionals. The roles of the different members of the team in caring for the patient and for the caregivers are described, as well as the multiple types of therapy and assistive technologies that are involved. The cost of these services is considered, along with sources of financial assistance through private insurance and government programs. Proactive approaches to legal matters including a living will, durable power of attorney, and other advanced directives for when the patient is no longer able to participate in decisions are described. Next, we will consider the impact of caring for a loved one with ALS on the family and friends.

7

Effects on Family and Friends

ALS is a disease that involves the patient, immediate family, and their social network in an intense and grueling struggle. Due to the current lack of effective disease-modifying therapeutic interventions, the process is suffused with an unavoidable level of hopelessness. Because of the nature of the disease and its progressive loss of function, much of the day-to-day caregiver role is shouldered by the spouse or significant other and often includes members of the immediate family and special friends. The patient also experiences much of the same stress, with the additional trauma of suffering the symptoms of the disease leading to the end of their life. In the previous chapter, the focus was on the long-term prognosis for the patient, planning for living with ALS, and organizing care. In this chapter, the emphasis is on the impact of the symptoms and their management on the psychological, practical, spiritual, social, informational, emotional, and physical needs of the caregivers and the patient's family and friends.

CAREGIVERS

The management of ALS is most effectively handled by a multidisciplinary team of health care professionals. For a variety of reasons including finances, personal preference, and geographical location, this level of care may not be available, or it may not be acceptable for all ALS patients and their families. Some patients are cared for in a medical facility, sometimes specifically designed to care for patients with a progressive physically debilitating disease. Many more are cared for at home, assisted by home visits from health care professionals, or they are brought to medical clinics by caregivers for assessments and treatments.

In either case, in addition to the burden of time and effort, caregivers are subjected to a number of psychological challenges. A family member, most often the spouse of the patient, becomes the primary caregiver, a role they were never professionally trained for, which causes them to be particularly susceptible to physical and mental stress and strain as they try their best to fulfill the role of caring for their loved one.

Caregiver burnout is a consequence of the intersection of a number of factors causing them to impose often-unreasonable demands on themselves. These include confusion, because the relationship between the patient and the family member changes as they are thrust into the role of caregiver. Unrealistic expectations of the caregiver in the face of a progressive fatal disease and a general lack of control over money, resources, and the skills necessary to plan and organize patient care are also factors.

Psychological Impact

The psychological impact includes many emotional components that combine to disrupt the regular experiences of life and affect the quality of life for both the patient and the caregivers. We all have certain expectations about what a normal life ideally should consist of. This may be briefly interrupted but usually resumes with minor changes after a particular crisis is resolved. With ALS, the life experience and those expectations take an unimaginable turn for the patient, which takes a toll as well on the caregivers and the family.

Accepting Diagnosis

Because arriving at an accurate diagnosis (see chapter 5) of an incurable disease like ALS requires the elimination of multiple treatable diseases with similar symptoms, diagnosis is arrived at by exclusion of those other possibilities. The still poorly understood mechanisms causing ALS (except for the familial forms) require further progression of symptoms in order for clinicians to be more certain of an ALS diagnosis. In early stages of the disease, there is often the hope that a treatable ALS mimic is the cause of the symptoms. Competing with this is that early treatment, symptomatic though it may be, can ease the symptoms for the patient.

Acknowledging and accepting the finality of the diagnosis is hard for both the patient and the caregivers, who face a difficult road ahead dealing with increasing disability and eventual loss of a family member. They often ask themselves questions such as, what brought this tragedy on the patient? What could they have done to prevent it? With our current state of knowledge, the answers to these questions are not obvious.

Anger and Frustration

Due to the increasing burden of caring for a progressively more disabled patient, it is not unusual for a caregiver to experience a degree of resentment with the situation. Although it may be suppressed, being forced to reconfigure their life and to have to deal with a disease for which there is no cure and with a prospect of only short-term survival for a loved one produces a fusion of both anger and frustration at the situation. The unpredictable progression of patient disability, with its series of plateaus and sudden declines, further stresses caregivers. Their feelings generally are not directed at the patient. The caregiver strives to keep feelings under control, or at least not visible to the patient, which produces a level of stress that makes the caregiving role more difficult.

Exhaustion

The sense of always being on duty and the psychological weight of being responsible for the first-line response to changes in the patient's status at any time of day or night can drive a caregiver's feeling of being overwhelmed. Physical exhaustion can also contribute, as the caregiver strives to be constantly alert and to stay ahead of the situation. Lack of caregiver sleep or the inability to fall asleep will take a toll on stamina, setting up a vicious cycle that makes the caregiver less able to render the care that they want to and to feel even more pressure to provide proper care. Asking for help seems to them to be an admission of failing in their role of taking care of their loved one.

Lost Intimacy

The stress and the responsibility of being the patient's primary caregiver take a toll in an especially painful way for the caregiver. As a spouse or other family member, they have a special personal connection with the patient that a professional caregiver does not share. They have shared life experiences with the patient, often amounting to several decades, which gives them special insight into the way that the disease and functional decline affect how the patient feels about their relationship.

Frequently, in order to personally function effectively, the caregiver has to establish a barrier of sorts, to set aside for the moment at least some of those thoughts and normal human reactions that a spouse or family member would have toward the person they had lived with or as a relative. This is a normal response that protects the caregiver to function in this stressful situation. Stepping back, figuratively, naturally results in a loss of a certain amount of intimacy in the caregiver-patient relationship. A key step in this process is for both the caregiver and the patient to be able to hang on to as much of their relationship as is feasible in the times ahead.

Clinician effectiveness relies on being able to put a certain distance between themselves and the patient that they are treating in order to focus on balancing what they need to do to best treat the condition while remembering to also serve the person who is their patient. This is part of their training and that of professional caregivers. Nonprofessional caregivers do not have this training and may not be able to achieve this level of separation.

Uncertainty about the Future

Because the condition of the ALS patient can change suddenly for the worse in different directions, caregivers feel unsure about how they will handle the next crisis that presents itself. Strategies for dealing with this ambiguity vary with the individual. It is important for caregivers to remain positive about their ability to rise to the challenge with the assistance and advice on call from the professionals on the case in order to show the patient that the changes will be under control. The positive attitude is also helpful for the caregiver to avoid becoming trapped in a downward spiral of confidence that generates additional stress and makes them less effective in their role.

Stress

The pressure that the caregiver is under is twofold: as the primary day-to-day caretaker and often as the spouse or a family member of the patient. It also comes from a variety of different angles or directions, each of which can affect the caregiver and their ability to care effectively for the patient. By identifying and watching out for the impact of some of these stresses, the professionals and clinicians of the management team can help the family caregiver to remain effective.

Caregiver Parental Relationship to the Patient

Although the average age of onset for ALS is mid- to later middle age, a significant number of patients have living parents. In addition, the age distribution of patients includes individuals who for a variety of reasons, genetic susceptibility or exposure to environmental risk factors, are considerably younger than the average ALS patient. In some cases, these parents take on a caregiver role for their now-grown child, with ALS as an extension of their former child care role. The patient may not have a spouse or other younger family members who want to or are able to take on the caregiver role. As might be imagined, this is a particularly difficult situation for a parental caregiver, who may not be in the best physical, financial, or mental shape to take on the formidable challenges of caring for an ALS patient. If possible, employing a paid or professional caregiver at least part-time would alleviate some of the stress while respecting a parental desire to care for their offspring.

Caregiver Working Status

At the time they become caregivers, many spouses are still employed in the workplace. Loss of income and medical coverage by both the patient and the caregiver puts many families in tough financial straits. Some spouses were career professionals who had to put that career on hold while they dealt with the family crisis. The financial and insurance repercussions add a layer of worry for the caregiver, in how caring for the patient will be paid for. While some employers will hold a position for an employee in this situation or have disability programs, in other cases the caregiver will lose their job. Those who were self-employed are especially vulnerable.

Caregiver Passive Coping Style

Individuals deal with stress in different ways. For some people, stress that is apparent to everyone around them seems to have minimal effect on them. The key point here is that it *appears* not to have any effect on them. More likely, they have some way of coping with the situation that is not outwardly apparent. Although it could be as simple as ignoring the stress until it comes to a crisis and then dealing with it, it also can simmer and build up pressure on the individual until they cannot handle it anymore and everything breaks down. The person can also be handling the pressure well, their different ways of coping not apparent to those around them. For those who are not coping with the situation, there are subtle signs of building pressure that trained professionals can discern. Again, this is something that the professionals and clinicians of the management team can help the caregiver with to remain effective.

Caregiver Symptoms of Anxiety

Anxiety is another way of describing worrying. Caregivers, of course, worry about the patient and whether they are doing a good enough job.

Being vigilant is important, but second-guessing every possibility and always assuming the worst-case scenario doesn't necessarily guarantee the best results. It is not useful and can even paralyze the caregiver when they need to make a decision about what to do in a given situation. Besides the mental anguish, physical symptoms of anxiety can be present, including uncontrolled trembling, heart palpitations, sleeplessness, even sweating and overall tiredness, leaving the caregiver listless. Not just the patient care suffers, but general day-to-day life is disrupted. Caregiver burden, depression, and anxiety are related and can be relieved by social support from others.

Anxiety is triggered by the fear of the unknown, of uncertainty, and of the lack of control of the outcome. Thinking about it will not solve the potential difficulty unless the caregiver can come up with an alternative, more likely scenario. It is possible to learn how to control and reduce anxiety. One way of dealing with this uncertainty is for caregivers to ask themselves how worrying about this will help and how will it hurt. Adopting an approach to minimize the damaging effects can help the caregiver weather the uncertainty. Anxiety can be exacerbated by triggers such as caffeine, sugar, and alcohol.

Perceived Quality of Care for the Caregiver

Caregivers need care too. As the disease symptoms in the patient increase and the disease progresses, the patient becomes ever more dependent on their partner, who is often the informal caregiver, as well as on other family members and friends. Care of the patient requires a great deal of time and effort on the part of all these individuals. Caregivers' strain and psychological distress increases as the disease progresses, due both to the increasing effort required and feeling the weight of responsibility for managing the patient care, which includes supporting patient decision-making and advocating for the patient. All of this leads to a worsening of the caregiver quality of life and a perception that they are not getting the support they need.

Patient Functional Status and Emotional Status

As the disease progresses and the patient's functional abilities decline, the burden on the caregiver increases. More and more of the patient's daily needs and activities require attention and assistance from the caregiver. This increases the strain on the caregiver both because of how intense the need for assistance is and how more profound the patient's deficits become. In addition, worsening function is a constant reminder of the approach of the terminal phase of the disease, triggering the beginning of the grieving process for the impending loss of the loved one. The need for interventions designed to protect the caregiver becomes sharply more acute at this point.

The emotional status of the patient also has a strong influence on the pressure felt by the caregiver. Even if the patient is not experiencing the emotional and cognitive functional effects of frontotemporal dementia, which afflict that significant fraction of ALS patients with cognitive or behavioral symptoms, the advancing ALS disease process changes the way patients perceive themselves and their relationship with others. This, in turn, impacts the caregiver, who may feel some responsibility for that perception. The patient's experience of losing independence and being locked inside a body that is increasingly unable to participate in even the most basic activities is bound to affect anyone's state of mind and the way they relate to other people.

Need for Caregiver Relief and Support Services

Caregivers report that identified shortcomings of management of an ALS patient's care were often due to the strain they were under. A number of both cross-sectional and longitudinal studies have identified a lack of interventions for alleviating caregiver strain. Currently, both ALS treatment guidelines and the ALS literature do not generally provide interventions to reduce caregivers' adverse experiences or caregiver strain. Studies are continuing to address these deficiencies, with the intention of providing guidance on appropriate interventions for the caregivers. The solutions are not likely to be simple, such as bringing in additional help, because, paradoxically, often neither the patient nor the caregiver wants or is willing to accept outside services.

While there is adequate information indicating a need in ALS management for specific effective interventions to relieve caregiver stress, exactly what they should include has not been established. There is a paucity, especially in the United States, of properly designed and sufficiently statistically powered studies that test potential interventions to protect caregivers in ALS. Because the medical care systems in different countries offer different levels of support and due to the relative rarity of ALS compared to other diseases, more studies focusing on the special challenges of ALS in the United States are needed in order to develop a consensus set of interventions.

FAMILY AND FRIENDS

Besides the patient and the caregiver, other family members and their friends are also strongly impacted when a patient is living with ALS. For 2–3 years or for some as long as 5 years, they all will be dealing with a fatal disease that is progressively and relentlessly debilitating for the patient, who will require more and more assistance. Obviously, the most dramatically affected are the patient and the primary caregiver. The first part of this chapter focused on the challenges facing these two individuals. For each family member, the impact will vary, depending on the involvement of that family member in providing day-to-day care for the patient, supplying resources, financial or otherwise, and taking on roles to take over the caregiver's part in the family operation to keep it running as smoothly as possible. Friends can provide helpful support at times or in situations where a family member is not available, or just as someone giving a helping hand when they see the need. The impact on the friend depends on the depth of the relationship among the friend, family, and patient and the extent of involvement in the care of the patient.

Psychological Impact

The initial symptoms of ALS are often not evident or a cause for worry even to the patient, unless they have been sensitized to the possibility because other family members have suffered from the familial genetic form of the disease around the same age. Only after a primary care physician picks up on the progressive worsening of the spectrum of symptoms that can present in ALS, refers the patient to specialists, and a diagnosis is sought does the possibility of ALS begin to sink in.

Accepting Diagnosis

For family and friends, the ordeal often begins during the diagnosis process. Suspense and anxiety build, as the testing proceeds over many months and multiple visits to medical clinics. Upon receiving the diagnosis, the patient and the caregiver, often a relative, are the ones who have to decide how and when they will communicate the news to other family members.

Informing children and elderly parents about the diagnosis requires special care, and this should be kept in mind when planning when and how to explain what will be happening to the patient and describing what the future will look like for the patient and the family. Children, especially young children, will require age-appropriate explanations of what will be happening with their loved one as the disease progresses as well as reassurance that they cannot "catch" ALS from the patient. Young children will need to be coached on interacting with the patient, especially in later stages of the disease when the patient can no longer respond verbally or physically but is still connected emotionally to the children.

The most directly affected family members are the immediate family, the closest relatives, especially those living with or nearby the patient and caregiver. These are the individuals who are most likely to be called upon to help with caregiving and transportation to appointments, to provide respite for the main caregiver, to take over roles the caregiver was active with in the community, and even possibly to help financially.

Anger and Frustration

Those adult family members called on to provide care or other kinds of support may experience resentment at interruption of their lives. This inevitably conflicts with their feelings for their loved one, producing anger and frustration with the situation. The extent of these feelings depends on the closeness of the relationship and the involvement with patient care. The potential for exhaustion depends on how much the family member is involved with patient care or caring for the caregiver.

Lost Intimacy

For family members who are not the primary caregiver but who are involved in patient care or in substituting for the caregiver in other activities, the pressure is not as intense as for the primary caregiver. It is nonetheless disheartening to watch the patient decline. With advancing functional decline, communication with the patient becomes more difficult, and it feels to the family members like the patient is shutting them out. It can be difficult for family members who are a step removed from the level of caregiver to realize that the lack of engagement on the part of the patient is the disease speaking, not the patient, who may be craving the interaction with family members.

This effect is magnified for friends, who may feel that they don't want to be a further burden to the family and the patient and may instinctively pull back from interacting. Strong friends will persevere in their support of the family and the patient, unless or until the family or the patient indicate that it is a burden to them.

Uncertainty about the Future

As for the caregiver, the plateaus and sudden downs of the disease progression create ambiguity for family and friends. Holding on to a positive attitude day by day will give confidence to the caregiver and patient and will help them the most in navigating the course of the disease.

Decision-Making

Two major mileposts in the progression of ALS involve the changes in respiratory function as the muscles of the diaphragm weaken. For most patients, they occur after a long string of debilitating losses of muscular control. Because they signal the final phase of the disease, they force the realization that it is time to decide on the lengths to which the patient wishes to go in order to prolong an ever more difficult life. In an ideally managed case, the decision about using assisted ventilation to extend life will have been taken earlier in the disease progression, after diagnosis and after the impact of what that verdict meant had a chance to sink in. That choice should also have been made while the patient would be able to make this kind of decision, especially in ALS-FTD cases, in which decision-making can be impaired.

Noninvasive Ventilation

The ability to modify that decision for breathing assistance remains with the patient, who may change their mind after having lived through the harrowing progressive loss of function and the fear of being trapped in a body that cannot communicate with the outside world, unable to make their wishes known. The first level of support, noninvasive ventilation, does not require major surgical intervention, but for the patient who realizes that this only postpones the inevitable, some just want it to be over. Many patients choose noninvasive support; fewer choose to go the route of major surgical intervention with a tracheostomy, which may give them a few extra months of survival.

End of Life: Withdrawing Support

The really agonizing decision is when to decide to let the disease take its course and not to prolong the suffering of the patient and the ordeal of the caregivers and family. Family members and friends may feel that they should not give up, but this is a decision that the patient and the caregiver have to be comfortable with, given the alternative of prolonged patient suffering that heroic measures would entail. This does not mean that family members and friends step away. Full support of the decision by family and friends, both of the patient and the caregivers, is needed for the final stage of the disease.

Concern about Genetic Heritage

Because ALS exists in both sporadic and familial (genetic) forms, it is natural for family members who are linked genetically to be concerned about the possibility that they are at increased risk for developing ALS. Familial forms can be identified by their early onset. Overall family genetic composition also increases the risk of ALS, as does the exposure to a common environment and experiences. Testing of family members for fALS genetic modifications and risk factor genes can alleviate some of these concerns. However, many people resist this type of genetic testing for ALS. They would rather not know, since having the genetic defect doesn't mean that the individual has a 100 percent chance of disease occurrence. The incidence of cases of the sporadic form of ALS vastly outnumbers the incidence of the familial forms. Having a family member with ALS increases the statistical risk of ALS occurring in the family, but it is by no means a certainty.

Coping with Stress

Like other health-related crises when the life of a loved one hangs in the balance, dealing with the practical and emotional impact on family members and friends is difficult at best, devastating at worst, for the individuals involved. In ALS, the most that can be hoped for is for the patient to experience the least amount of suffering. To reduce the stress on family members and friends, different family members employ a variety of coping strategies. The effectiveness of each approach depends on the individual. What works for one person may fail to reduce the stress for another person. It may very well require multiple approaches applied simultaneously or different approaches at different stages of disease progression to weather the situation.

Adopting a Problem-Solving Approach

The trajectory of ALS is marked by a series of events that occur over the not-always-continuous decline in patient function. Foreseeing and identifying difficulties as they arise and focusing on solving or alleviating those specific issues are a practical way for family members and friends to feel that they are contributing to some measure of control of the situation. A feeling of helplessness builds stress.

Living Day-to-Day

Not looking ahead too far, especially with a terminal disease like ALS, is another coping strategy. Dealing with the here and now focuses on what can be done at present to support the patient without being overly concerned and therefore anxious over what looms in the future.

Trying to Remain Positive

Having a positive attitude about what is currently being done for the patient and how the immediate future looks is good for the patient, caregivers, and family and friends. This is not an effusive, overly positive outlook, but a perspective that looks for and emphasizes positive aspects of the situation. It is all too easy to fall into negative thinking about the prospects, and such thinking can be contagious. This helps no one.

Inhibiting Signs of Grief to Appear Strong

It is important to realize that, regardless of how it appears to people on the outside, caretakers, family members, and friends of a patient with ALS are all grieving the impending loss of the person they care about. They express this in different ways and with different intensities. To avoid causing the patient distress over the effect of their illness on family members and to project support for the care plan, other family members and friends often suppress negative feelings, not letting them show. Feeling despair while displaying a positive attitude is a source of stress for family members and friends and is an important component of the grieving process.

Changes in the Meaning of Life

If anything positive can come from the experience of being a family member of a loved one who died from ALS, it is the recognition of the important things in life. Not everyone will have this reaction. Many are unable to view the events as anything other than a horrible experience. Those who are able to reflect may derive some sense of closure and achieve a new perspective on who they are. The exact meaning often differs between individuals, but there are also common themes. They can become maturer, stronger, and more appreciative of the little things, and as a result, they can become more involved in their own life experience. They feel lucky and privileged to be healthy or are thankful that an illness they do have isn't a death sentence. Their principles and values have been tested and may have changed, and they now have a better grasp on what is important to them.

Having a family member with ALS causes a great deal of stress and psychological anguish for others with a close relationship with the patient. The burden is particularly heavy for those who have taken on the mantle of caregiver. This chapter considered the support needed by the caregiver and by the other family members, relatives, and close friends commensurate with their level of involvement with the patient and the caregiver. Next we will consider how this disease could be more rapidly and specifically diagnosed and its causes better understood in order to develop strategies for effective treatments that prevent the disease or slow or halt progression.

8

Prevention

In order to prevent a disease, it is necessary to understand enough about how the normal functioning of the complex mechanism of the human body begins to go wrong in that disease. It is quite natural to feel that when someone displays symptoms of an illness, the causative event happened recently. When a child catches a cold, she very often remembers that the boy behind her in English class yesterday was coughing and sniffling. But many other diseases take much longer to develop than the common cold. The initiating event could have happened long ago or more recently and just wasn't noticeable.

In order to develop strategies to prevent the illness or stop it from progressing, the instigating process and/or the sequence of events before the symptoms are noticeable have to be identified and understood. Only then can interventions like a vaccine, an antibiotic, changes in lifestyle, or protection against exposure to certain environmental conditions become effective. At our present state of understanding, the early stages of ALS are silent to the individual, and no reliable biomarkers have yet been identified until the symptoms appear. By the time the patient notices the diagnostic muscle weakness, the disease process is already well advanced, and functional decline proceeds rapidly. Therapeutic measures at this stage so far have, at best, added only a few months additional survival.

PREVENTING A DISEASE WHOSE ROOT CAUSE IS UNKNOWN

For a disease like ALS, it is difficult to approach prevention when the root cause(s) are unknown. While it is thought that there is a multistep progression to the first symptoms, the individual steps remain to be defined. There is a lack of specific, reliable biomarkers or signs of ALS prior to symptoms of any of the steps that can warn of the future. The accumulation of insults or stresses does not seem to occur in any particular order, and what may be a stress contributing to the progression for one person may be innocuous in another individual. There is no indication of the approach of the tipping point that will lead to motor neuron dysfunction or muscle-degeneration-producing symptoms, their spread, and the ensuing functional decline.

Prevention for a disease in which the causative process(es) are unknown begins with efforts to delay disease progression as well as to alleviate symptoms and promote function. One logical approach has been to start with an animal model of a familial form of ALS where an individual's genetic mutation is a strong initial insult that likely starts the disease process very early. Investigators can then work to find interventions that lengthen survival and slow the loss of function, which then can be tested in human clinical trials. This has been the main approach to date.

Strategies for Delaying Symptomatic Disease in At-Risk Individuals

The presently most reliable way to identify ALS at-risk individuals is through establishing a history of ALS in a lineage of genetically related family members. Genome analysis tests for the presence of one of the current 29 or more genes mutated in ALS. It can also check for combinations of other gene variants or mutations that significantly increase the risk of ALS when they occur together. Genetic predisposition often leads to a somewhat-earlier age of onset of symptoms, but even this is not an absolute predictor for ALS. There are a significant number of individuals with a genetic predilection for ALS who, even when they reach middle age never develop the symptoms or functional decline. They may have sustained a subthreshold level of the damage to motor neuron or voluntary muscle systems typical of ALS, but never progressed in severity to the symptomatic stage.

Faced with a genetic predisposition, it would be logical and appropriate for the genetically at-risk individual to avoid exposure to the suspected environmental, occupational, and lifestyle risk factors that don't necessarily cause ALS by themselves but can contribute to progression to symptoms. Once ALS symptoms appear, the instigating damage has already occurred, leading to spread of the weakness to muscles connected to the neuronal pathways that, in most cases, eventually undergo rapid functional decline. In a few individuals, for reasons that are not understood, functional decline can slow dramatically, and they live longer before the final stage, where the respiratory muscles succumb.

Slowing Symptomatic Decline

Effective symptom management (covered in chapter 5) and supportive care provide better quality of life for individuals with ALS. Unfortunately, supportive measures have been primarily palliative. They don't measurably slow the rate of decline of functionality, which actually accelerates as the disease progresses, increasing to an exponential decline when respiratory function becomes impaired. In the United States, the two FDA-approved therapeutics for the treatment of symptomatic ALS, edaravone and riluzole, which work by different mechanisms, have been of limited effectiveness. Edaravone actually showed a measurable slowing of the rate of functional decline, but the study trial was not powered to determine whether survival time was affected. Riluzole, on the other hand, increased survival time by several months.

Clinical trials most often compare patients who are already symptomatic for their response to the drug or a placebo. While it might be possible through such trials to demonstrate a therapeutic effect, there is a very good chance that the damage has already been done and the cascade activated. Dead motor neurons are not replaced, and any therapeutic effect is likely to be small. Preventative trials treating patients who are not yet symptomatic will require much more complete understanding about what causes the disease. It will also involve the identification of predictive biomarkers for some of the steps in the process to judge efficacy. This latter point is where we would like to be.

IDENTIFICATION OF AT-RISK POPULATIONS

With a relatively rare disease such as ALS (worldwide prevalence less than 5 in 100,000 persons) researchers have to find a sampling method called a *study design*, to increase the odds that a sufficient proportion of the people recruited into a study group will actually develop ALS. Researchers need to identify people who have a greater chance because of a strong risk factor of developing ALS than the overall population. They must also identify a group of people who do not have that risk factor for comparison. From what we know now, the identifiable individuals most at risk are those with a family history of ALS.

Genetic Risk

Currently the only practical measure for selecting a study group for ALS is to follow the genetic risk, the strongest and most reliable link known to the disease. A small percentage of the people who have ALS (5–10 percent) inherited a gene mutation that predisposes them to ALS. Some of these are familial mutations that cause ALS in a high proportion of those gene mutation carriers. Individuals with certain mutations in the genes for particular proteins present symptoms at a somewhat-younger age than those lacking a genetic susceptibility. Importantly, the age of onset for these individuals is more predictable for each mutation of a gene, because symptom onset tends to cluster around a particular age for that mutation, unlike those with nongenetic forms of the disease (sALS), who show a broader and older age distribution.

Other individuals carry mutations in one or more genes other than the familial ALS genes. When those mutant genes are present together in the same individual, that person's risk of developing ALS is increased. These persons are considered to have a genetic predisposition to ALS, but not all individuals will progress to symptomatic ALS. Their genetic risk is less severe than those with familial mutations. By studying these people at genetic risk of ALS identified by genetic analysis of their DNA, researchers have a much better chance of defining the beginnings of the disease process that eventually lead to symptoms. The incidence of ALS is also affected by race, where a common pool of gene variants contribute a genetic component; some of these genes as a group can result in an increased (or decreased) incidence of ALS. Ethnicity, although technically not a genetic risk factor, can influence incidence in a population by promoting standards of cultural behaviors that expose the individual to increased (or decreased) risk of developing ALS.

Genetic Testing

Genetic testing for ALS is focused on the detection of mutations in a specific gene or genes and is performed to determine whether a currently asymptomatic individual in a family with a history of ALS has inherited the mutant form of the gene. This is a diagnostic test one might think akin to a diagnostic glucose-blood test. However, since the entity (a gene) tested for in ALS carries implications for other individuals in the same generation as well as for future generations, there are stricter ethical standards applied to doing the genetic test at all, as well as to the rights of the patient with respect to disclosure of the results. A more detailed explanation of the process is provided in chapter 5.

Genetic screening is different. It is often requested by an individual, and performed by a commercial company, in order to look for the presence of known mutant forms of disease-associated genes where there is not necessarily a family history. Many companies offer this testing. It is the responsibility of the individual being tested to be aware of their rights and the extent of their control over the use of the information.

We next will consider the issues and controversies that are at the heart of the ALS field limiting its progress in understanding the disease and in developing therapeutic treatments that slow or block progression.

9

Issues and Controversies

As a disease without a cure at this point in time, ALS is confronted by multiple issues and beset by a number of controversies. This wealth of uncertainty does not mean that the problems are unsolvable. We are early in the process of understanding what causes the degeneration of the nerve-muscle circuitry, what factors lead to vulnerability of certain individuals, how we can detect early signs, and, of course, how we can stop or even cure the disease at a stage where the individual experiences minimal dysfunction. A number of other diseases originally faced similar barriers to progress, and perseverance and innovation was able to overcome them. Still others, also neurodegenerative diseases, remain largely untreatable except palliatively, although in a significant number we are learning how to recognize their early stages. This chapter will delineate the key obstacles facing the medical and research communities in resolving the controversies and addressing the issues hindering progress in diagnosing and treating ALS, as well as in delivering effective care and support for ALS patients and their families.

ISSUES

The biggest issue for the ALS community is the lack of therapeutics that can effectively preserve patient function over an extended period of time by slowing the time course of disease progression. It is clear from the many trials of potential therapeutics run in small patient cohorts that there is likely no "magic bullet" that will stop ALS in its tracks or return a nonfunctioning patient to normalcy. Sensitive assessment measures are required to confidently observe an effect over a brief time, because after diagnosis, ALS progresses so rapidly. Also, because ALS is a relatively rare disease with rapid progression, assembling a large-enough group of ALS patients to obtain results that aren't due to chance can be challenging. Finally, there appear to be multiple forms of ALS, beyond the broad familial (genetic) and sporadic classifications, which further complicate trial design.

Even though we have recognized ALS as a disease since Charcot gave it a name in 1874 and know quite a lot about the disease, we still do not have a solid handle on presymptomatic diagnosis in a time frame and stage of the disease where we have a good chance of affecting its progression. Nor do we have a detailed overall understanding of what is going on in the patient as the primary disease process driving progression as opposed to a peripheral secondary effect.

ALS is not alone in this relative lack of understanding of the primary forces driving the disease process. Multiple, major age-dependent neurodegenerative diseases affecting millions of people, including Alzheimer's disease and Parkinson's disease, face many of the same issues. Frontotemporal dementia affects numbers of individuals, 60,000 in the United States, closer to the 20,000-case prevalence of ALS in the country. A major difference is that there are much better presymptomatic measures of the disease progression for these other neurodegenerative diseases, than for ALS although we still only have palliative treatments for them.

Only Hint of ALS Is the Presence of Symptoms

A major issue is that the only reliable indication of ALS for diagnosis is the set of physical symptoms of the disease, even though they are not individually unique to the disease. There is no blood test, imaging, or other biomarkers that conclusively and specifically identify ALS and distinguish it from a number of other disorders, some of which are treatable. Even voluntary muscle function tested by electromyography is a relatively late manifestation of the disease. In addition, the development of the presymptomatic changes is slow, age dependent, and unrecognizable as ALS, compared to the progression of the symptomatic phase of ALS, leaving little opportunity for effective intervention after diagnosis. The relative rarity of ALS compared to other diseases with similar symptoms but with different or more benign consequences also impedes accurate diagnosis.

In some cases, genetic analysis can identify known familial forms of ALS, due to mutations in particular proteins that track in families.

However, that only identifies potential disease status often but not always associated with increased risk of developing ALS. For these cases, the age of onset of symptoms is younger and only relatively predictable. This uncertainty is because disease expression is also influenced by multiple other genes, by environmental and other risk factors, and by different combinations of these elements. The apparent multistep progression to symptom appearance is a consequence of these interactions.

Lack of Diagnostic Biomarkers for Presymptomatic ALS

Diagnosing ALS is a lengthy process, especially with respect to the rapid time course of the symptomatic and functional decline phases. It is presently one of exclusion, ruling out other diseases with ALS-like symptoms. Although differences in muscular function and nerve conduction can be detected by the proper technology, they aren't symptomatic (not necessarily noticed by patients) and frequently don't predict when symptoms will appear. More molecular markers are being studied. Unfortunately, for practical reasons, many of these markers are tied to the familial forms of ALS, because the familial form of ALS can be predicted to develop the genetic form of ALS, although they account for a small proportion of all ALS cases. At this point, it is not clear yet, despite the similarities in loss of muscle and neuronal function, that all or even many of the changes that occur in familial ALS will also occur in the much more common sporadic (nongenetic) form of the disease.

Identifying common pathways and their changes prior to physical symptoms linked with the amounts and types of molecular components present in easily accessible biofluids will go a long way toward improving diagnosis. Early diagnosis will lead to earlier treatment and a better opportunity for interventions to have a substantial effect on disease progression and maintenance of function.

Lack of Disease-Modifying Therapeutics

Development of effective therapeutics to treat ALS has been hampered by the inability to rapidly diagnose the disease, stemming from the lack of diagnostic biomarkers that are sensitive to the earliest stages of the disease process before symptoms are noticed by the patient. This, in turn, is the outcome of an insufficiently complete understanding of the disease process, which hinders the ability to reliably detect presymptomatic changes early enough in the disease process to know when and where to intervene effectively.

The root of all of the delay in diagnosis is the complexity of early disease processes, which is now being recognized as being due to a multistep disease process (see chapter 8) in which multiple hits affecting key processes mount up to finally overwhelm normal protective mechanisms. While the currently approved drugs address some of the mechanisms thought to be driving the disease, their effects on improving function, slowing disease progression, or in extending patient survival are relatively minor. Clearly there is more going on than we currently understand, in part because by the time ALS is diagnosed, it is too late, as too much damage has already been done to the motor neurons and the voluntary muscles they control.

New lines of research are being designed to reach out and apply the effects of the mutations found in human familial ALS cases. Since fALS mutations were the only situation where researchers know that ALS would result, this was the starting point for using model systems including genetically modified mice producing the human mutant protein. An example of these new studies is the focus on human cells cultured from stem cells isolated from ALS patients. Stem cells can be from either familial or sporadic cases, which gives researchers the opportunity to learn about the similarities and differences of the types of disease under different conditions, including treatment with materials believed to be active components triggering disease progression caused by environmental exposures, for example. These models may also be useful for testing new therapeutic interventions.

Delivery of Care

In addition to the scientific and medical issues identified above, there remains the thoroughly practical problem of ensuring that the individual patient receives the appropriate level of care in the optimal time frame regardless of their financial situation. Although many diseases and their management are complex, ALS is especially challenging because it is not only extremely difficult and time-consuming to diagnose but it also lacks truly effective disease-modifying treatments. It is a very rapidly progressing disease with an average life expectancy of about 30 months post diagnosis. Many patients have a shorter survival. There is little time to waste getting into active treatment.

Because the disease is so complex to deal with, it requires a multidisciplinary approach (see chapter 6) and a team of professionals coordinating care in conjunction with the caregiver, often a family member, at home or on site with the patient. Efficient coordination between members of the team and communication with the patient is essential, as are ready access to clinic appointments, transportation to appointments or home visits by team members, and timely availability of assistive technology. With so many moving parts and complex organization in practice, there are numerous points at which there is delay as the process is interrupted or communication is incomplete.

Health care systems in different countries all struggle with the coordination of diagnosis and care services for ALS patients, regardless of the level of central or government organization of medical care. In the United States, access to facilities able to deal effectively with diagnosing and managing the care of ALS patients across the country is geographically spotty, often requiring extensive travel, which becomes increasingly difficult for patients as they lose functionality. The relative rarity of ALS is also a factor here. Not every medical facility can afford to field a full set of ALS clinical specialists, because the patient population is too small.

Delivery of care for ALS patients remains a difficult issue that requires resolution. In the short term while effective therapies are being sought, the infrastructure for managing ALS can continue to be improved so that the system works more effectively.

CONTROVERSY

While there is scientific debate over which mechanism(s) drive the degeneration of motor neurons and the muscles they innervate in ALS, two questions could have the strongest effect on reducing the incidence of ALS: what are the risk factors and how do they exert their effect? Although the field understands that risk factors for ALS are a major driving force for the disease, a major controversy surrounds the effort to define how much of an effect the individual risk factors contribute, how they act in combination, and what accounts for differential effects among ethnic populations. Even some partial answers could be helpful in tracking down situations with the largest effect. This will be a difficult issue to address and to resolve. There are many opinions out there without conclusive evidence pointing one way or the other.

Role of Risk Factors in ALS

In order to resolve these issues, many unknowns need to be discovered. In addition, a number of observations coming out of studies of ALS incidence with respect to potential risk factors need to be convincingly assessed for their contribution to the ALS disease process. It has proven difficult to determine which factors contribute the most to the risk of developing ALS. Part of this is due to fact that, for the most part, the risks are what are termed *compound variables*, made up of a collection of individual toxic agents or stresses whose effects are individually and collectively hard to quantify.

Mixtures can have different effects, which may also depend on the age of the individual or ethnic or genetic heritage. Examples that have received a great deal of study and generated a comparable amount of controversy are environmental insults, lifestyle choices, and occupation, especially active deployment in military service. Because these are categories, each factor is multicomponent, variable in time of exposure, and broadly defined without good quantification. Only statistics of large groups of people are available, which are difficult to apply to the relatively small number of individuals who develop ALS.

A further complexity arises as it appears that the hits, disease-promoting events that can be simply risk factors, may not have to occur in a particular order to cause disease. Identifying these risk factors and assessing the magnitude of their effects has proven extremely difficult (see chapter 8). Susceptibility can depend on multiple parameters, and it has also been difficult to determine how exposure to the risk factors leads to the deficits seen in ALS. At present there is controversy over whether the risks are truly significant or only more apparent than real. Besides providing guidelines for limiting environmental and occupational exposure in general and in particular for individuals with identifiable genetic predispositions, learning how these exposures lead to ALS would aid in better understanding the disease process itself. It would also provide hints as to how to reduce their contribution to the development of ALS.

Contribution of Variants of Dominant Familial ALS Genes versus Nonfamilial Risk Genes

Genetic predisposition, most obviously in familial cases inheriting certain dominant mutations in proteins like SOD1, FUS, TDP43, and C9orf72, is the most potent risk factor for ALS, but these mutations only occur in about 10 percent of ALS cases. They cause early onset disease, somehow bypassing or reducing the contribution of the aging component of ALS, middle age for sporadic cases. There are also numerous genetic factors whose effects are subtler. They do not cause disease individually but act in concert with other gene variants to cause a normally innocuous exposure or experience to trigger disease mechanisms. DNA sequencing of these individual gene variants in the genomes of individuals is identifying an increasing number of interactions that end up influencing the disease process by interacting with risk factors in some way.

Contribution of Epigenetic Factors to the Genetic Component of ALS

One of the mechanisms that accounts for the observation that "DNA is not destiny" is epigenetics, a system analogous to software that controls the use of the basic coding potential in the DNA sequence. This is likely to be the level at which the risk factors operate on pathways that can lead to disease. A complex system, it is new science and thus is far from being understood in the detail required to make sense of all of the possibilities. The extent of these epigenetic changes is unique to the individual, and their effects can last a lifetime. While they are generally not passed on to the next generation, for reasons that are currently not well understood, modifications can persist into the next generation. In some cases, they can even cause certain traits to seemingly skip generations. Epigenetics and whatever other modulation of genetic potential out there could be key to finally understanding why certain people suffer ALS and others under similar circumstances fail to develop the disease.

The issues facing the ALS community are profound. Researchers still do not have a good picture of the causes and the development of this complex disease at its earliest presymptomatic stages. They do not yet have reliable clinical biomarkers of these stages to predict who will develop the physical symptoms that signal the inexorable and rapid decline of function. Currently available therapeutics fail to halt the functional decline.

While environmental and lifestyle risk factors are suspected and there is some evidence in support of these possibilities, there is considerable disagreement over what these factors do and how they cause their effects that lead to ALS. The strongest linkages seem to be at the genetic level, but less to the genetic code of the DNA and more at the level of when and how strongly the genetically coded information is expressed. This is controlled by an epigenetic process that responds to what the organism experiences, which may prove to be the target of the risk factors. The next chapter describes the current efforts of the research community to understand the disease process, find reliable markers, and develop new and effective therapies.

10

Current Research and Future Directions

There is presently a tremendous flurry of research activity pursuing the causes, risk factors, biomarkers, progression, management, and therapeutic strategies for ALS. Stimulated by the influx of funding and momentum derived from the crowd-sourced Ice Bucket Challenge, which carried over into renewed interest by NIH, ALS research is now punching far above its weight in research interest. The death on March 14, 2018, of the theoretical physicist and longtime ALS patient Stephen Hawking woke the world up. He had survived almost complete paralysis from ALS for over five decades, defying the normal survival times of 3–5 years post diagnosis. It reminded us that we still have neither a preventative strategy nor a cure for this disease. At the same time, his long-term survival extended hope to ALS patients that *something* allowed Hawking to survive so long. It give support to the idea that it should be possible to intervene in the so-far-inexorable progression and to prevent functional decline and death.

This chapter describes ongoing efforts to tackle treatment of ALS at multiple levels. It includes defining and understanding the presymptomatic changes in the patient that, to this point, have been invisible. By dividing the process into addressable stages, it may be possible to locate and define the tipping point at which the normal physiological function of motor neurons and muscle fibers begins to degrade. With these parameters delineating the presymptomatic phase of the disease, the early stages of the rapid symptomatic phase, that occur before massive neuromuscular degeneration causes dramatic functional decline, can then be approached. Biomarkers for this phase could be used to speed the currently rate-limiting diagnosis of ALS, generating the precious interval to test potential therapeutics in order to intervene early in the apparently downhill process once symptoms appear.

Clinical trials continue to test drug therapeutics. Researchers are also now moving into considering stem cells and their products along with types of genetic manipulation approaches. These include proof-of-concept interventions targeting fALS with highly specific tactics directed at the mutant gene.

SEARCHING UPSTREAM: PREVENTION, THE EARLIEST PATHOBIOLOGY, AND THE SEEDS OF ALS

Because of the combination of the overall rarity of ALS, the current multistep disease model predicting multiple hits that add up to progress to the clinical disease, and the unknown order in which those stages can occur, it is difficult to formulate the kind of straightforward, logical approach available for many other diseases. It is even hard to collect a large-enough patient group for meaningful study. For these reasons, a practical approach to finding an effective treatment for ALS is to start with the known risk factor with the largest effect on the probability that a person (or a model organism) exposed to that risk factor will develop ALS.

As described in detail in chapter 8, the largest and most predictable risk factor for ALS is genetic, specifically those dominant mutations in C9orf72, SOD1, FUS, or TARDP = TDP43 protein genes, which account for 60–80 percent of familial ALS cases. There are 25 or more other genes linked to ALS in families, but they are distributed among the remaining 20 percent of fALS cases. In fALS patients, *all* cells in the body contain the mutant gene and thus are potentially exposed to its effects from conception.

Novel Biomarkers and Outcome Measures

Improvement and validation of biomarkers for use in ALS diagnosis and therapy development is a major aspect of current and future ALS research. Biomarkers indicate different aspects of a disease state useful for detecting disease, following progression, and evaluating effects of treatments in clinical trials for therapy development. Some can be diagnostic for the presence of the disease; others can be predictive of which patients are likely to respond to a particular therapy, and still others are prognostic of future progression rate.

Examples of biofluid-derived biomarkers currently being validated for clinical use in ALS include the light-chain form of a neurofilament protein, which is a structural protein released from dying neurons, whose concentration increases in cerebrospinal fluid during ALS progression. Levels of urate, also found in urine, and as a metabolic waste product in the blood are decreased during the course of ALS, instead of the increases seen in a number of other diseases. A specialized immune cell type called a *regulatory T-cell* decreases in the blood in rapidly progressive cases of ALS. These tests and others under development are expected to provide earlier answers during diagnosis and to monitor disease progression that is not immediately functionally or symptomatically apparent.

Not only proteins have the ability to serve as biomarkers of disease. A small but very special type of ribonucleic acid molecule called a *microRNA* (miRNA), discovered in 1993, was found to regulate gene expression by blocking the production of specific proteins or blocking other RNA molecules that have other functions in the cell. Of particular interest is that a number of the genes connected with ALS, such as FUS and TARDBP = TDP43 protein, play a role in RNA processing pathways, including the biogenesis of these miRNAs. In addition, multiple forms of human ALS are characterized by an overall reduction in the amount of miRNAs.

MicroRNAs are found in many biological fluids (blood plasma, cerebrospinal fluid, tears, and saliva), and changes in the levels of different miRNAs can be linked to different cell types. Widely used in cancer research to distinguish different types of cancer, ALS researchers have been working to exploit the miRNA changes in ALS patients to classify patients, monitor disease progression, and predict patient response to potential therapeutic interventions. They also are comparing animal models to human patients in order to look for similarities, to identify potential therapeutic targets, and to determine mechanisms. The goal is to be able to diagnose earlier and more accurately, perhaps even well into the presymptomatic phase, to start treatment. Incorporating miRNAs into biomarker analysis for ALS is currently underway and making progress.

THERAPY DEVELOPMENT

The National Institutes of Health, in addition to a number of private and nonprofit organizations, sponsor research to find new targets, develop more predictive animal models, and test innovative approaches to treating ALS. A small percentage of the research will progress to development of potential therapeutics and testing in humans in clinical trials. Clinical trials are expensive and require very careful consideration of their design to be able to interpret the data, because the magnitude of the improvement, also known as *effect size*, of therapeutics in ALS trials has always been small. A multitude of ongoing clinical trials of varying trial design are testing potential therapeutic treatment strategies for ALS; for examples, see https://www.als.net/als-research/als-clinical-trials/#. Some exciting new tools are being developed to better understand human ALS, and they perhaps will provide unanticipated therapeutic options.

Looking Ahead in ALS Therapy Development

A 2017 review described the results of advanced (phases two and three) randomized controlled trials testing efficacy of potential therapeutics for ALS. Fifty-one clinical trials were completed, testing 25 different compounds representing 10 broadly different mechanisms of action. The trials reviewed were performed and reported on by industry and academia between 1995 and July 2016. These trials, each enrolling more than 100 subjects for adequate statistical power, totaled 13, 427 ALS patients and used the Revised ALS Functional Rating Scale (ALSFRS-R) to measure efficacy. Although ALS animal-model studies showed significantly large enough effects to propel these test compounds to clinical trials, effects of these potential therapeutics on the human disease were minimal.

These studies included riluzole and edaravone, the only treatments that showed a significant impact on patient functionality. In addition, patient selection for the edaravone clinical trial run in Japan was only in Japanese patients and was highly selective, only enrolling a narrow segment of patients with certain characteristics representing as few as 1 in 20 of the type of patients being followed at an ALS clinic. For regulatory agencies, this limits the applicability of the results to other patient populations. Expanded patient populations are being planned for edaravone, and impact on survival will be evaluated. Of particular future interest to patients, an oral formulation of edaravone is being developed to replace the more invasive intravenous infusion delivery of the current dosage form.

A variety of antiglutamatergic, anti-inflammatory, antioxidative, neuroprotective, and neurotrophic growth-factor therapeutic agents were tested in randomized controlled clinical trials. They addressed a variety of mechanisms of supporting motor neurons in particular, as well as other cell types in the brain, spinal cord, and muscle. In addition to riluzole and edaravone, only an antineuroinflammatory, masitinib (Masivet® [for veterinary use]), a specific inhibitor of certain tyrosine kinase enzymes that has received orphan drug status in the United States and Europe to target cellular inflammation responses in ALS, met a primary end point of the study. It demonstrated a significant functional effect and slowing of progression in combination with riluzole. Further trials of masitinib are underway and seeking FDA approval.

If approved as safe and effective, its oral-dosing regimen could improve patient compliance over edaravone delivered by infusion.

STEM CELL THERAPIES

One of the difficulties in using animal models of ALS to understand the human disease is that mice are not humans. Researchers have taken a step toward addressing this concern by using skin and other cell types easily obtained by biopsy from individuals with ALS as a source of inducible stem cells. These are unspecialized cells that can be caused to develop into specific types of cells that carry the genetic complement of that individual, mutations and all. Applied to inducible stem cells from both fALS and sporadic ALS patients, the similarities and differences can be compared after differentiation into other cell types, such as motor neurons or muscle cells. This may help researchers learn why therapeutics that were effective in an fALS mouse model failed in human trials.

The low number and small effect size of current pharmacologic therapeutics for ALS emerging from clinical trials has opened the field to sophisticated nonpharmacologic-based therapeutic approaches. In the body, and particularly in the brain and elsewhere in the nervous system, the many different types of cells work together as a community and produce materials needed by other cells. In ALS, multiple cell types are affected by the disease, not only motor neurons and the voluntary muscle cells that die during the course of the disease. As a result, critical growth factors and regulators that reduce inflammation and other toxic processes may be lost or inappropriately expressed, causing dysfunction in the motor neurons and muscles. Therapeutic approaches that provide replacement cells that can respond to the diseased environment by producing the deficient materials could remedy the situation.

Stem cells are unspecialized cells present in many body tissues that are capable of developing into multiple other cell types. They act like internal repair centers, responding to changes in their environment by dividing to produce new cells that develop (differentiate) into cells with different properties and functions. Current stem-cell approaches aim to provide cells that will produce growth factors and other protective factors to support motor neurons rather than try to replace dead motor neurons.

Mesenchymal stromal cells are a kind of stem cell isolated from fat or bone marrow biopsies. They are derived from the ALS patient, grown up in culture, and injected into the patient's spinal cord or muscle, where they differentiate to express the neural genes in order to provide the growth and other protective factors that the damaged motor neurons or muscle cells need to survive. Immunosuppression, often used in transplantation to avoid rejection, is not needed here, because these are the patient's own cells. Researchers have developed ways of treating the cultures, some including genetic modifications that induce them to produce larger amounts of the needed factors. Currently, only small-scale clinical trials, enough to test for safety, have been performed in ALS patients, but some reports indicate that a subset of patients may be responding.

Another approach, injecting stem cells generated from neuroglial precursor cells from fetal embryos left over from in vitro fertilization into the spinal cord, has been used in small trials. Since the stem cells are not from the patient, immunosuppression is required to prevent rejection of the transplant. Again, modest but encouraging effects were observed in a subset of patients, and larger multicenter trials are being planned.

Research using human-patient-derived stem cells differentiated into motor neurons or muscle cells to test therapeutics is expanding. While this work began with familial ALS cases as the source of stem cells, it is now recognized as a way to study the much more common sporadic form of ALS and to compare therapeutic strategies.

Personalized Medicine: What's New in Therapeutic Approaches

Human-patient-derived biopsy cell samples can also be dedifferentiated to another kind of stem cell: *inducible pluripotent stem cells* (iPSCs). As their name indicates, these precursor cells then can be reprogrammed to redifferentiate into motor neurons by adding appropriate growth factors and differentiating agents. Gene editing to repair a familial ALS mutation in the iPSCs before redifferentiating them into motor neurons can theoretically also be undertaken. A new method employing CRISPR/Cas9 gene replacement has been used to accomplish this with high fidelity in iPSCs in culture. The same methodology applied to a human patients and directed specifically to motor neurons remains to be optimized and validated for specificity and tested for off-target modifications. In humans with the CRISPR/Cas9 genetic manipulation, additional ethical considerations and controversy would need to be resolved before moving the correcting of mutations line of research into humans.

ANTISENSE OLIGONUCLEOTIDES AND RNA SILENCING

In familial ALS where the mutated gene is known, a strategy is to target the production of that particular protein. This can be done with agents that specifically recognize and cause the degradation of the precursor message, which would normally be translated into protein by the cell. This strategy is currently being applied in several neurodegenerative diseases. A series of separate clinical trials are employing agents called *antisense oligonucleotides*, which are specific for the individual diseases delivered into the cerebrospinal fluid. This approach is being developed to treat Huntington's disease, ALS-SOD1, and Alzheimer's disease.

For ALS, antisense oligonucleotides to SOD1 have thus far demonstrated safety in humans in early clinical trials, and ongoing studies are planned to study efficacy. An antisense oligonucleotide strategy has been shown to be effective against another genetically driven neurological disease, spinal muscular atrophy, in clinical trials. The drug, nusinersen (Spinraza), has recently been approved by the FDA, and a similar treatment, eteplirsen (Exondys 51), for Duchenne muscular atrophy has received conditional approval.

C9orf72-associated ALS is the most common familial form of ALS. C9orf72 is a gene containing multiple repeated sequences whose number of repeats tends to increase in families over generations. These expanded numbers of repeats in the message cause them to accumulate and inactivate important proteins in different cell types, causing cell death. Treatment of C9orf72 mouse models with antisense oligonucleotides has alleviated C9orf72-dependent adverse events, setting the stage for human clinical trials.

CAUSES FOR OPTIMISM

Successful treatments that affect progression of the disease and especially survival, even if suboptimal, offer the opportunity for deeper understanding of disease mechanisms in ALS. This is because they identify and impact rate-determining pathways in the disease process. With a handle on these pathways, researchers can backtrack into the driving forces, look for measures that can be used as biomarkers, and judge their specificity for ALS. At the same time, as effective therapeutics are being discovered, disease pathways and mechanisms can be determined and even more effective treatments developed.

Case Illustrations

TOM

Tom, a 60-year-old man undergoing his yearly routine physical, explained a nasty bruise on his knee to his primary care physician, saying that he had tripped on a stair step. He was trying to improve his physical fitness by climbing the stairs at work to his fourth-floor office rather than taking the elevator. Catching the toe of his right shoe on the edge of a step made him stumble, but he mostly caught himself on the stairway railing. Upon questioning, Tom admitted that over the last few months, he was also having trouble with his footing when playing tennis, part of his reason for exercising more.

The internist examined the right foot. There was no external sign of an injury, and there was no pain. Compared to the left foot, the patient had trouble lifting the front of his right foot from the ankle, and the right foot wouldn't support walking on his heels with the fronts of his feet elevated. Since it was possible that the weakness was due to spraining the foot, the internist asked him to come back later to check to see if the weakness had resolved.

The weakness was no better a week later, and it was diagnosed as *foot drop*, a neuromuscular condition that can be a symptom of many different diseases. Since no hip replacement, knee-ligament reconstruction surgery, stroke, or diabetes with its generalized peripheral neuropathy was involved, these conditions sharing the same symptoms could be eliminated from consideration. The remaining list of possibilities, though, was daunting: spinal disk herniation, stroke, muscular dystrophy, multiple sclerosis, Guillain-Barré syndrome, Charcot-Marie-Tooth disease, and ALS. At the local hospital, Tom began seeing a neurologist, who initiated a full physical and diagnostic workup. Over the next several months, diagnostic immunological testing was negative for Guillain-Barré syndrome, and genetic testing failed to find evidence for Charcot-Marie-Tooth disease, which also mostly strikes younger individuals.

As time passed, the weakness in Tom's right foot intensified and spread to adjacent leg-muscle groups. Tom was finding it harder and harder to climb stairs at work and finally gave it up, because of worries about falls. Regular neurologic exams were performed to assess the progression of the disease. The spreading nature of the muscle weakness to other muscle groups connected by the same motor neuron pathways was highly suggestive of ALS. The results of diagnostic testing had ruled out a number of look-alike neuromuscular diseases, or at least made them appear highly unlikely. Diagnostic magnetic resonance imaging ruled out some other causes, and testing nerve conduction and the electrical activity of muscles in the affected regions confirmed the increasing dysfunction.

By a process of exclusion, the diagnostic team was closing in on a diagnosis of probable ALS. They then turned to diagnostic tests that would identify the ALS disease variant involved in order to estimate progression and survival time. There was no evidence in Tom's accessible family that other family members had inherited the potential for ALS, but the patient agreed to genetic testing, which was performed in case he might have developed a gene variant whose identity might predict the disease progression.

Finally, the diagnosis of ALS was communicated to Tom and his family, along with what they could expect about the disease course and what it would mean. A plan for management and treatment and identification of resources for his care and the family caregivers was worked out. Genetic counseling was provided in additional sessions to inform family concerns about possible shared genetic potential for ALS, especially for Tom's children. The diagnostic process required many months of stress on Tom and his family, but their early detection of the problem will at least allow them time to prepare for the ordeal.

Analysis

The symptom of foot drop is a relatively common, although not the only initial, presentation for ALS. Fortunately, this patient's primary care physician didn't put off investigating the implications of what started out as only a minor inconvenience. The diagnosis of ALS is burdened by a lack of specific biomarkers for the disease, which results in a protracted set of studies that are mostly exclusionary, ruling out other potential diseases, some of which have viable therapeutic options. In lieu of biomarkers, progressive loss of functionality is used as a surrogate to indicate that the disease driving the changes is ALS. The workup is thorough and includes genetic analysis and counseling to inform family members of their genetic potential to develop ALS, which is a major concern of families.

Identification of resources and the presentation of a management plan are designed to assist families in dealing with this interruption in their life. The standard of care for case management is through a multidisciplinary team approach that takes advantage of trained professionals to support the primary caregiver(s), who handle much of the day-to-day patient care. This support can be critical for reducing stress in the caregivers.

JILL

Jill, a 50-year-old woman from a rural farm family, visited a neurologist at her regional hospital, complaining of recent, lingering mild neck and shoulder weakness following exercise. Her concern was that she had two male relatives, a brother and a cousin in their late forties, who had both died after being injured in separate, similar machinery-related accidents where leg weakness, lack of coordination, and stumbling were factors. Although there had been essentially no medical follow-up on the cause of the accidents, Jill's neurologist suspected that the cases might be familial ALS, because there were other family stories about similar incidents. Although Jill's relatives' accident circumstances suggested lower limb involvement rather than her upper body weakness, Jill's neurologist suggested testing for genetic factors that might be involved.

His suspicions were justified when the lab results showed that Jill carried one normal copy of the SOD1 gene and one copy of an A4V mutation in the SOD1 gene. This mutation was dominant, with one copy of the mutant gene sufficient to cause ALS. This particular mutation is the most common familial ALS cause in the United States, involved in 50 percent of all U.S. familial ALS cases involving SOD1, which account for 10–20 percent of all fALS cases. Although fALS represents only 5–10 percent of all cases of ALS (sporadic and familial), the genetic dominance, relatively early onset, and range of survival outcomes are more predictable, but also more extreme.

For Jill, the most important implication was that the A4V mutation is an extremely aggressive form of ALS. Onset of disease symptoms is sudden, and the time courses of disease progression and functional decline are extremely rapid. Survival time after symptom onset for A4V SOD1 is 17 months, compared to 30 months for sporadic ALS, little more than half as long.

Jill was understandably stunned. The weakness seemed so minor, yet the functional tests the neurologist ordered indicated that the dysfunction was already spreading. She was now worried that other people in her family needed to be warned about this genetic monster stalking their family. The case manager explained to her how genetic counseling protected patient family members who may or may not wish to learn their genetic status with respect to ALS. The case manager also outlined the limited counseling and support services available in Jill's region to help her to cope with what was happening to her.

Jill and her husband operated their own farm in a rural, isolated farming community served by a regional medical center with a long-term-care facility. They decided that the long-term-care facility would be best able to provide her with care, as neither of them had any medical experience. Her husband wanted her to be close enough for him to visit often. He would be struggling, even with the help of neighbors to manage the farm on his own. Lacking the income or private insurance to cover all of the bills for this incurable disease, the couple was mostly relying on local community social services.

The long-term-care facility was not experienced in coping with the range of disability that Jill would bring to them. Because ALS is relatively rare, they had never cared for a patient with ALS before. They would have to learn with long-distance input and borrowed equipment from the nearest ALS clinic, which would also send a staff member with ALS expertise to evaluate and advise the team in the rural long-term-care facility every few months.

This was not an optimal solution, but it was the best one available under the circumstances. Jill and her husband were consulted at every step and would do their best to make it work.

Analysis

Recognition of the potential for a genetic connection in this case and thus a familial contribution to what turned out to be A4V SOD1 fALS was important. Despite the female gender of the patient and the prevalence of the A4V mutation in males (A4V 1.3:1 males:females) and initial bulbar symptom presentation instead of the more common lower limb onset, this case was rapidly diagnosed, instead of wasting valuable time waiting for more typical ALS symptoms to appear. This was a critical outcome that put this rapidly progressing subtype of ALS in perspective in order to plan for its sudden changes and the extraordinarily rapid time course of functional decline.

The isolated rural location of the patient's residence and single-family farming occupation constrained the opportunities for optimizing long-term care for ALS. This was the result of the couple's preference for the husband to be close enough to visit while still operating the family farm, as well as the need to rely on local social services to provide medical care. The local long-term-care facility lacks experience with ALS care but visits, consulting, and equipment have been arranged with a more distant ALS clinic. While not an optimal solution, it provides for the basic care for the patient using local resources in line with their wishes and situation.

ROB

Rob, a 40-year-old male, was experiencing muscle weakness in his left and right shoulders and upper arms that had progressively weakened over a period of 2 years without noticeable spreading to muscles of other limbs. After a series of tests, he was surprised by a diagnosis of an atypical form of ALS called *flail arm syndrome*, also known as *man-in-a-barrel syndrome*. The cause of the differences from the classical limb type of ALS, which involves the legs and arms, or the bulbar type, which affects the muscles of the face, jaw, and throat, is not well understood. A major difference from classical ALS was that Rob was expected to live for up to 5 years, maybe even longer. The final outcome would be the same with slow spreading of weakness, eventually to the lower limbs and to the diaphragm, compromising breathing.

As a relatively young man with a family, Rob had to work to wrap his head around this prospect. As his kids were growing up, he would be increasingly unable to participate in their lives. Rob was fortunate that his office job provided adequate medical insurance coverage for ALS. After discussing the situation with his wife, he made the decision to go on disability early, because he wanted to be able to be with his family while he could still could do some activities with them for as long as practical. They arranged to manage his care through an ALS clinic in a local hospital. His wife was going to be his main caregiver, but she would be aided by a health care team providing guidance and clinical support.

At first, Rob enjoyed being at home and the center of attention. He could still walk, although the lack of strength in hands, arms, and shoulders increased the possibility of a head injury from a fall, because he would be unable to use his hands and arms to support and protect himself. Initially, physical therapy with active and passive exercises maintained his mobility and functionality. He was able to do most small things by himself. So far, he had avoided the painful contractures by keeping the weakening muscles moving.

Rob was, however, becoming frustrated by his clumsiness and increasing inability to use his hands for the simplest self-care tasks, such as fastening buttons, tying his shoes, or dressing himself. Even getting in and out of bed, or sometimes simply using a chair, became a major effort. Finally, he had to ask for help with what had always been simple things. At this point, he also began using devices specifically designed for ALS patients recommended by his health care management team. Simple splints to support arms and hands and devices that harnessed what muscular control remained to him gave him the ability to control his range of motion. Rob's loss of hand strength and coordination made it difficult for him to communicate by handwriting, typing on a computer keyboard or tablet, or using a cell or landline phone.

He was able to use special splints with grips designed to help with holding implements for writing and utensils for eating. Rob was especially eager to learn about eye-gaze technology so that as his disabilities increased, he could use it to control devices and to communicate. Being restricted to a wheelchair would be coming at some point, but that didn't bother him so much. At some point, he was likely to lose his ability to speak. The possibility of becoming "locked-in" for years, to function mentally normally but to be unable to make his wishes known or to respond to his family, was always on Rob's mind. He wanted to be prepared.

Analysis

This ALS patient's unusual presentation of symptoms frequently could lead to misdiagnosis as one of a number and variety of diseases including carpal tunnel syndrome, multifocal motor neuropathy, spinal muscular atrophy, or even a herniated disk. The proper diagnosis spared the patient the ordeal and expense of additional testing and perhaps some unhelpful or possibly harmful treatments designed for different disease processes.

The extended timescale of the disease progression and the slower decline of function in flail-arm syndrome compared to classical ALS allow patients more time to cope with the changes that inevitably occur as disability increases. This patient with a young family chose to be with them while he still had functionality. By engaging with a health care management team at a local ALS clinic soon after diagnosis, he was able to put himself in the best position to maximize the functional time with his family. Losing the use of hands and arms early on in the disease course, before the process begins to involve the legs, provides additional challenges for the caregivers, but the slower progression will allow for adaptation. Assistive technologies will be needed over a longer period to contribute to patient safety and ability to do for themselves. Further enhancements of this equipment to better support patient functionality are still needed.

RACHEL

Rachel, a 65-year-old woman with progressive lower limb muscle weakness, was diagnosed with classical ALS. Her family and her management team were proactive in accommodating her increasing physical disability at her home. As she became more restricted in her ability to perform simple tasks for herself, the patient began to be easily frustrated, breaking down crying and becoming angry, at first only with her caregivers. This behavior from a no-nonsense woman who had always controlled the expression of her emotions surprised her caregivers, who did their best to soothe her. They rationalized her behavior as a reaction to being diagnosed with an untreatable terminal disease. Why wouldn't someone be angry with such a prognosis? Soon Rachel began to also have difficulty finding words to express herself, a behavior that didn't fit with what her caregivers had been told by her neurologist to expect from someone with ALS.

Rachel's neurologist explained to the caregivers that recent studies had established that 15–50 percent of patients initially diagnosed with ALS also showed signs of a variant of *frontal temporal dementia*. FTD affected emotional processing and language deficits like word use as well as executive functioning affecting judgment and decision-making, inhibitory control, and motivation. Fortunately, dementia itself, which affects many other types of behavioral and cognitive function much more severely, was not usually seen in patients with ALS. Cognitive and behavioral screening tests have been specifically developed for use in ALS patients whose physical limitations affect their ability to respond. Two tests, the ALS-Cognitive Behavioral Screen and the Edinburgh Cognitive and Behavioral ALS Screen, would help predict the impact of the cognitive and behavioral changes on the management so that the care team could prepare for the unique challenges presented by the confluence of ALS and variant FTD in the patient.

Rachel was evaluated by both diagnostic schemes, which differ in their sensitivities for detecting cognitive and behavioral deficits, and was diagnosed to have ALS-FTD. The care management team immediately began to consider how to handle the unique challenges this diagnosis presents, since overall evidence-based guidelines for ALS-FTD management have not been established. One of the first chores was to establish her wishes in writing with regard to medical decisions while Rachel was still cognitively able to make decisions. This included when, or if, to implement respiratory assistance (noninvasive/invasive) when that stage of the disease was reached. It also included what to do about end-of-life decisions in the terminal stages of the disease. The early diagnosis gives at least some time for those involved to come to terms with the eventuality that, at some point, Rachel will be unable to effectively take part in some decisions.

Analysis

Her caregivers' recognition of the patient's unusual emotional lability soon after her ALS diagnosis was important. Their follow-up with the

clinical side of the management team was a key factor in the early deter-
mination of the coexistence of ALS and FTD in the patient. It gives the
case management team some much-needed extra time to prepare for the
additional burden contributed by the FTD disease component. In particular, having the patient make her wishes known about medical decisions
while she was still judged mentally competent was critical. This also
applies to making important legal decisions in other matters, such as set-
tling her estate. Often these considerations can fall through the cracks
when dealing with caring for the patient. Most important for the patient
are the decisions involving noninvasive and invasive respiratory options
and end-of-life-stage interventions.

Early identification of the cognitive and behavioral component also provided time to prepare the caregivers and the family for the additional physical and emotional burden imposed by the FTD component on top of the
life-threatening ALS disease process. This included supportive counseling
for family members and for regular respite time and psychological assistance for the caregivers, especially the primary caregiver.

The fact that many behavioral clinics are not set up to deal with the
physical disabilities inherent to ALS also impacts case management.
The cognitive and behavioral impairments are certain to negatively impact
the management of the continuing physical decline. Understanding that
Rachel's behavior is caused by the FTD part of the disease can help the
family cope with the behaviors. Symptomatic treatment with antipsychotic
drugs to control agitation or aggression may be helpful in alleviating some
of the symptoms. Issues of judgment and patient compliance will also be
affected by the FTD.

There is no effective treatment for either the ALS or the FTD part of the
disease process, although riluzole may provide some survival benefit in
ALS. Survival time of patients with ALS-FTD does not differ significantly
from those with ALS. The burden on the primary carer is significantly
increased in ALS-FTD, due to the added behavioral and cognitive
complications.

JIM

Jim, a 62-year-old male veteran of the First Gulf War, had been nursing
a sore leg for a few months that had suddenly reappeared, reminding him
of his injury from jumping out of a helicopter when his unit was engaged in
a firefight during the conflict. That injury had put an end to playing first
base in baseball's minor leagues, although no one would guess that he had
a problem with fitness these days. His activity in the workplace and strength
and endurance in physical activities showed no hint of his war injury.

Jim could put up with the inconvenience of a flare-up of the old injury, but what was now worrying him was that the other leg was starting to refuse to respond when he tried to move quickly. Like all budding baseball players, Jim had heard of Lou Gehrig and the strange neuromuscular disease that robbed him of his strength, coordination, and ultimately his life. He decided not to say anything to his family yet, but the thought nagged at him. When he went to his primary care physician to get therapy for the sore leg, he waited until the doctor had his hand on the examining-room doorknob, ready to leave, to ask about the weakness and lack of pain in the other leg. Was it Lou Gehrig's disease, ALS?

There was good reason for Jim to be concerned. He had two of the main recognized risk factors for the disease outside of a genetic predisposition. He was athletic and fit, and he had served in the military in active combat in a war zone. Several anxious months and a seemingly unending series of tests at a Veteran's Administration clinic that specialized in neuromuscular conditions later arrived at diagnosis of classical sporadic ALS. In the interim, Jim had worked through the initial shock of being diagnosed with an incurable rapidly progressing disease. Jim's first concern was for his family. How would they fare during the course of his increasing disability and then without him? Right up front was the issue of how they would be able to afford the cost of his care.

The U.S. health care system is a complicated hybrid of government and private sources of support and services that requires planning to access effectively, especially for a disease with a rapid progression. Not every individual qualifies for all of the benefits, so sorting this out early is a priority. Because he was a U.S. veteran, Jim had access to VA hospitals through his VA benefits. Since military veterans are recognized to be at increased risk for ALS, the VA gives guidance and has resources dedicated to the disease. Jim's ALS diagnosis qualified for VA disability, which he had to apply for. Benefits would be retroactive to the application date, but processing would take time. In addition to social security benefits, diagnosis of ALS qualifies for Medicare Part A and Part B, although Medicare Part B requires a separate application.

Private medical and other insurance, such as that he obtained through his employer, provides coverage that will help fill in the gap until the government programs kick in and will help pay for expenses not covered by the government programs such as modifications to a residence to accommodate wheelchair use, or hospital-style beds and lifting devices. The appropriate private medical insurance can help with these expenses.

Nongovernmental organizations, such as local ALS Association chapters and the ALS Guardian Angels, offer advice in navigating the process of seeking support as well as helping families find some financial resources. They are also are sources of information on loans or least expensive options for medical equipment. Some individuals with ALS have resorted to crowd-funding tactics through Go Fund Me campaigns.

Analysis

Being eligible to access the resources of the Veterans Administration and the VA hospital system for medical care and advice is a valuable asset for this veteran with ALS. His anticipation of the possibilities tempered by the impediments of the system should stand the family in good stead. Knowing how to access and to use the system is important. However, administration by its huge, layered bureaucracy often causes delays, and administrative squabbles can try the patience and temperament of stressed families and caregivers, who are trying to deal with managing the often-erratic course of the disease and the prospect of watching a loved one suffer.

Arranging available financial support for care for the ALS patient early in the progression of the disease is important for limiting the damage to the family's financial future. Losing track of or putting off these arrangements until later disease stages, when there are increased stress and responsibilities on caregivers involved with the patient, can make for hasty and unsound decisions. In addition, getting approval for government support and benefits can have long processing periods or have built-in delays after approval before eligibility starts. There are few compromises built in for diseases such as ALS with rapid progression.

Glossary

ALS–Clinical Functional Rating Scale (ALSFRS)
A clinical rating scale for ALS based on activities of daily living and respiratory criteria.

Aspiration pneumonia
Pneumonia initiated by choking and inhaling saliva and food, causing a lung infection.

Atrophy
Shrinking, withering. In ALS, this generally refers to muscle wasting.

Biofluid
A fluid from the body, such as blood, urine, cerebrospinal fluid, saliva.

Biomarker
An objective, quantifiable physical feature or molecules that are associated with a particular disease state.

Body Mass Index (BMI)
A calculated measure of body fat based on adult height and weight.

Bulbar ALS
A form of ALS that initially affects muscles in the head, face, neck, throat, and mouth, primarily affecting swallowing chewing and talking. Motor neurons in the bulbar region of the brain (hence the name) are the first affected.

Clinicopathological
Signs and symptoms directly observable by a physician and those found in laboratory tests.

Cognition
Acquiring knowledge and understanding through experience, sensation, observation, and thought.

DNA (deoxyribonucleic acid)
Genetic material of the cell that encodes the information for producing all of the cellular components.

Durable power of attorney
A person you appoint to act in your place for financial and other purposes. *Durable* means that this person continues to act in the event you become incapacitated. This distinction is important, because other types of power of attorney cease when you die or become incapacitated.

Dysarthria
Disorder due to weakness or defective muscle control of speech, causing slurring, slowness, and poor pitch control.

Electrodiagnostic
Measurement of nerve and muscle electrical activity.

El Escorial criteria
A diagnostic scale designed for research purposes combining clinical observations with electrophysiological measurements of nerve and muscle function.

Epigenetic
Changes in gene expression that are not dependent on DNA sequence of the gene.

Ethnicity
Sociological factors (culture).

Excitotoxicity
Damage to or killing of nerve cells from overstimulation by neurotransmitters, such as glutamate.

Executive function
Brain involvement in decision-making, planning, strategizing, motivation, and being able to control responses (inhibitory control).

Familial
Tending to occur within a family of genetically related members more often than by chance.

Fasciculations
Spontaneous muscular contractions and relaxations or twitches.

Fibrillation
Uncoordinated contractions or twitching of individual muscle fibers within a muscle.

Flail arm variant
Variant of ALS characterized by initial severe wasting and weakness of arm muscles without involvement of other body regions.

Flail leg variant
Variant of ALS characterized by initial severe wasting and weakness of leg muscles without involvement of other body regions.

Foot drop
Difficulty in lifting the front part of the foot. Usually a symptom of a greater problem.

Free radical
A highly reactive but generally short-lived molecule that chemically combines with and damages biological systems.

Frontotemporal dementia
A group of uncommon brain diseases that affect regions of the brain responsible for controlling personality, behavior, and language.

Gene
A physical and functional unit of heredity encoded in an ordered sequence of DNA (deoxyribonucleic acid) units.

Glia
Nonnerve cells in the brain that perform a variety of functions to support the nerve cells. Typical glia are astrocytes, microglia (immune function), and oligodendroglia (insulation of neurons).

GWAS (genome-wide association study)
A study of the association (connection) of genes with biological or biomedical functions or diseases. *Association* suggests involvement with and possible causation.

Human genome
Complete set of the DNA sequences present in the 23 human chromosomes, including protein coding and nonprotein coding DNA sequences.

Incidence
The rate of new cases of disease per 100,000 population over a time period, usually a year (see *prevalence*).

Innervation
Connection of nerves with a target.

King's clinical staging
Clinical rating system following the spread of the disease that focus on the number of body regions affected. It is most sensitive to changes early in the course of ALS.

Lower motor neurons
Neurons in the spinal cord and brain stem that receive signals from upper motor neurons and pass on their signals to lower limb muscles.

Magnetic resonance imaging
An imaging technology used to visualize soft tissues such as the brain. It is not sensitive to the earliest changes in ALS that result in symptoms, so in general it is not useful for early stage diagnosis but can detect other non-ALS-related changes.

Metabolic activity
The chemical reactions in the body that provide energy to drive cellular functions and building blocks to make new cells and molecules controlling cellular interactions.

MicroRNA
Small ribonucleic acid molecules that regulate the activity of expressed genes.

Milano-Torino functional staging
Measures the burden of dysfunction and is most sensitive in later stages of ALS.

Motor cortex
The part of the cerebral cortex of the brain that initiates the activity of voluntary muscles.

Mutation
A change in the DNA sequence of a gene.

Nasalgastric (NG) tube
Flexible tubing inserted through the nose and passed through the esophagus into the stomach.

Neuron
A specialized cell designed to transmit information to other nerve cells, muscles, or glands.

Neurotransmitter
A chemical released upon stimulation by a nerve cell that crosses a narrow gap and produces an electrical response in a connected nerve, muscle, gland, or other structure.

Palliative treatment
A treatment that reduces symptoms and improves the quality of life but does not change the course of the disease.

PET (positron emission tomography)
In ALS, an imaging technique that uses a short-lived radioactive chemical to reveal metabolic activity or other function in the brain, nerves, muscles, and other organs in a patient.

Phenotype
The observable characteristics of an organism.

Presymptomatic
Occurring before symptoms are observed by the patient.

Prevalence
The number of cases still alive as a fraction of the total population at risk over a time period, often a year (see *incidence*).

Prognosis
Prediction of the likely development and course of a disease.

Progression rate
In ALS, the time between first symptoms and diagnosis.

Race
Biological factors, such as genetics.

Risk factor
A characteristic, attribute, or exposure of an individual that increases the probability of developing a disease.

RNA (ribonucleic acid)
An intermediate produced by the cell from its DNA sequence that is used by the cell to make the proteins that allow the cell to function.

Schwann cell
A glial cell type that wraps around neurons in the peripheral nervous system, providing an insulating layer to increase the speed of signal transmission. In the central nervous system, analogous glial cells, oligodendroglia, perform the same function for central neurons.

Sign
Objective evidence of a disease not felt by the patient, as opposed to *symptoms*, which are subjective because they are felt by the patient.

Sphincter
A ring of muscle that closes or opens body openings, such as the anus and in the stomach.

Stem cells
Unspecialized cells present in many body tissues that are capable of developing into multiple other cell types.

Symptom
Something a patient can feel or see related to a disease.

Synapse
A junction between two nerve cells or between a nerve cell and a muscle cell across which an electrical or chemical signal is passed.

Syndrome
A set of symptoms and signs that occur together, frequently associated with a particular disease or disorder.

Upper motor neurons
Neurons originating in the cerebral motor cortex of the brain or the brain stem. Some upper motor neurons innervate the face and neck; others transmit signals to lower motor neurons in the spinal cord, which pass on their signals to lower limb muscles.

Directory of Resources

ASSOCIATIONS

ALS Association
http://www.alsa.org/

ALS Society of Canada
https://www.als.ca/

International Alliance of ALS/MND Associations on the Internet
www.alsmndalliance.org

FOUNDATIONS

A Life Story Foundation
https://www.alifestoryfoundation.org/

ALS Foundation for Life
http://www.alsfoundation.org/

RESEARCH

ALS Clinical Trials
https://www.clinicaltrials.gov/ct2/results?term=amyotrophic+lateral+sclerosis

ALS Research Forum
http://www.alsresearchforum.org/

ALS Therapy Development Institute
http://www.als.net/

National Amyotrophic Lateral Sclerosis Registry
https://wwwn.cdc.gov/als/

SUPPORT

The ALS Residence Initiative
http://www.alsri.org/

ALS Support and Help Forum
http://www.alsforums.com/

Compassionate Care ALS
http://www.ccals.org/

Family Caregiver Alliance
https://www.caregiver.org/

BOOKS

Anderson, Peter. 2014. *Silent Body, Vibrant Mind: Living with Motor Neurone Disease.* Melbourne, Australia: Brolga Publishing.

Barkan, Ady. 2019. *Eyes to the Wind: A Memoir of Love and Death, Hope and Resistance.* New York: Atria Books.

Bromberg, Mark B., and Diane Banks Bromberg. 2017. *Navigating Life with Amyotrophic Lateral Sclerosis.* Oxford: Oxford University Press.

Butzer, Rosemary. 2017. *The Journey—The Mike Vollmer Story.* Self-published, Amazon Digital Services.

Caldwell, Sarah. 2015. *Just to Make You Smile: A Teenage Daughter's Reflections on Loving and Losing Her Father to ALS.* Boynton Beach, FL: Sedonia's Magic Words.

Dunsky, Eliot H. 2016. *ALS: An Orientation.* Self-published, CreateSpace.

Fitzmaurice, Simon. 2018. *It's Not Yet Dark.* Boston: Mariner Books.

Gollin, Michael. 2014. *Innovation Life Love: Reflections on Living with Mortality.* Self-published, CreateSpace.

Hawking, Stephen. 2013. *My Brief History.* New York: Bantam Books.

O'Donnell-Ames, Jodi, and Terry Heiman-Patterson. 2015. *Someone I Love Has ALS: A Family Caregiver Guide.* Gorleston, UK: Rethink Press.

Rymore, Robert. 2013. *Lou Gehrig Disease, ALS or Amyotrophic Lateral Sclerosis Explained. ALS Symptoms, Signs, Stages, Types, Diagnosis, Treatment, Caregiver Tips, Aids, and What to Expect.* IMB Publishing.

Selley, Richard. 2018. *Death Sits on My Shoulder*. Self-published.

Sherman, Casey, and Dave Wedge. 2017. *The Ice Bucket Challenge: Pete Frates and the Fight against ALS*. Lebanon, NH: ForeEdge.

Spencer-Wendel, Susan, and Bret Witter. 2014. *Until I Say Good-Bye: My Year of Living with Joy*. New York: Harper Paperbacks.

Swainbank, Dan. 2015. *The Farr Disease: One Family's 150-Year Battle against ALS*. St. Johnsbury, VT: Raphel Marketing.

Index

About the Author

Harry LeVine III, PhD, is associate professor in the Sanders-Brown Center on Aging at the University of Kentucky in Lexington, Kentucky. He is author of *Genetic Engineering* and *Medical Imaging*. A 28-year veteran of the pharmaceutical industry, his focus is on developing therapeutic approaches to age-dependent neurodegenerative diseases. He specializes in Alzheimer's disease, especially the protein-misfolding mechanisms that it shares with ALS.